A Place to Anchor

Journalism, Cancer, and Rewriting Mi Vida as a Latina on the Border

ESTELA CASAS

Contents

Who I Was

"Estela has such a beautiful voice!"

When I was a kid, I'd always dreamed of being a singer. I sang in the school and church choirs and for family and friends.

And even though it was far more expensive than she could afford, my mother arranged for me to have voice lessons.

Wherever it was, I sang, using the voice God gave me, confident in His gift.

But making a career out of singing just never happened for me. There are a variety of reasons for that, but I like to think it's because God knew my voice could do more than just sing. I wound up using my voice to help amplify *others'* voices, crafting myself a career in broadcast journalism as a storyteller.

In the newsrooms in which I worked, I advocated for "people stories." I gave up my right to a public opinion, choosing to be a "just the facts, ma'am" kind of journalist. I started my broadcast career as a part-time reporter at KTSM, the NBC affiliate in El Paso, Texas. News director Mike Malter saw something in me, and after a three-hour interview, I got my foot in the door. The first story I ever covered was about the new satellite dishes at the station.

In 1984, KINT, a group of business owners, decided to open up a Spanish language news station. I was one of the founding journalists, hired as the weekend anchor/reporter. Two months later, I moved into the prime-time anchor spot. I worked at Noticias 26 for a year, before being courted back into English language news at KDBC by General Manager Sam Kobren, news director Bill Mitchell, and anchor Al Hinojos.

I made my mark at the El Paso CBS affiliate with the Wednesday's Child segment on hard-to-adopt children, and the Texas Breast Cancer Screening Project.

I was at the anchor desk in 1985 during the earthquake in Mexico City that left more than 5,000 people dead. I went on air to tell our community that teacher Christa McAuliffe and six other crew members had died as the Space Shuttle *Challenger* exploded during liftoff in Cape Canaveral, Florida. I covered stories across the border in Ciudad Juarez, Mexico, on the murders of women and girls and the drug wars. I covered city council and commissioners court meetings, El Paso Electric and Texas Gas budget hearings, and rate increases. During my tenure, I also covered Fort Bliss's role in the Gulf War during Operation Desert Storm. In short, I did it all, with a focus on listening to, and giving a platform for, the community's voices.

After eight years with KDBC, I had the opportunity to move to the number one station in the market. I started at ABC affiliate KVIA with Gary Warner and Suzanne Michaels in 1993 as the 10 p.m. anchor/producer. I was behind the anchor desk during the terror attacks on the World Trade Center, September 11, 2001.

The highlight of this career? A five-minute interview with sitting president Barack Obama. I was the only El Paso journalist invited to talk to President Obama about the Trans-Pacific Partnership.

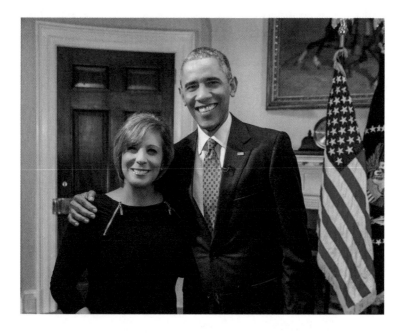

And as honored as I was to conduct that interview, I was just as honored to be able to share stories of education success with my Estela's Escuelas series, and with my monthly Keep Abreast segment, reminding women to perform regular self-examinations for breast cancer prevention. I shared many life events with

KVIA-TV viewers, including a high-risk pregnancy in 2002, my battle with thyroid cancer in 2010, and my journey with bilateral breast cancer in September 2017.

I was on a cattle drive the weekend a lone gunman drove hundreds of miles, walked into an Eastside Walmart with a machine gun, and sprayed it with bullets, killing twenty-three people and injuring dozens more. Those stories were some of the hardest to tell.

At that point in my life, I realized that reporting on two cancer diagnoses, and on the tragedies of others, had changed me. I had worked so long to amplify other people's voices, but I had somehow lost mine along the way. While telling a news story *can* be personal, it's not the same as opening the whole box of emotions around that story.

I began questioning my reason for being. Something in my heart and mind stirred, making me feel like I wasn't working with a purpose. I became restless, looking for my place in the world, trying to remember when I'd lost my fearlessness.

In 2015, I was a woman who was not afraid to ride a bike alongside semi-trucks near Portland, Oregon, for a marathon. But I'd since hung up my bicycle in the garage. I put away the clips, helmet, and padded shorts. I'd become afraid to start pedaling my way back, not just on the road, but also mentally speaking, to face life's challenges.

The road full of traffic ahead felt intimidating, fearful, and filled with doubt. I knew I had to make drastic changes to help bring back my fearless self.

I wanted her back.

I needed her back.

So, I began the journey of writing this book. Come with me, and see how cancer reminded me who I was, how it helped me reclaim the things it attempted to steal, and how it taught me to acknowledge that it's the simple things that reveal the greatest truths.

This is my truth. Esta es mi realidad.

CHAPTER ONE

Broken and Beautiful

Many things make me who I am.

I'm an orphan. I no longer have parents, or the stability of having the two people who both loved me unconditionally (while also being my harshest critics) just a phone call or visit away.

I'm the mother of three beautiful children: a girl, a boy, and a bonus baby. Despite having my fallopian tubes tied, cut, and cauterized, despite having a six-inch cut above my pubic bone to remove a large cyst inside my left ovary, I still got pregnant five years later! My son, Andres, was a fighter and an unexpected blessing then, and is a fighter and a continued blessing now.

I'm a sister to two brothers, and a sister-in-law to two exceptional women.

I'm the ex-wife to my high school sweetheart, to whom I was married for thirty-two years.

I am a BMAC—a beloved monogamous adult companion. (That's how I describe my significant other because I'm too old to call him my boyfriend.)

I am a friend to friends I can count on one hand. I'm a coworker and health advocate. I am a news anchor and journalist.

I am, through all of these, a woman. A tough, determined, strong-willed woman who fought her way through life and career, enjoying many successes. But when confronted with a diagnosis of synchronous bilateral breast cancer, it doesn't matter how strong you are, how much you are loved, or even if you feel you're living a seemingly perfect life. Hearing "You have breast cancer" takes your breath away!

Even though, as a journalist, I'd spent decades focusing on women's health, done countless stories on the importance of breast cancer prevention and research, and organized the very successful Texas Breast Cancer Screening Project as a news anchor at KDBC TV in El Paso, I felt overwhelmed and frightened by the diagnosis.

Twenty-five years ago, I did a special report on the importance of getting a mammogram. I don't remember a lot of the stories I've done in my almost four decades as a journalist, but this particular story stands out in my mind and in my heart. I recall that day in stark detail because it was life-changing. Little did I know that God was getting me a little uncomfortable, preparing me for my own journey.

The story covered my personal experience of having my first

mammogram. I wanted to do that story to show women that, "If I can do it, so can you." I was assigned a male photographer because we didn't have a female photojournalist on staff. Brent is a little older than me and is married with two beautiful daughters. He is mature, a great photographer with the talent to get the perfect angle, to show enough to know what's happening, while still making it appropriate for the evening news.

In the newsroom, Brent was making sure he had all the proper equipment for the delicate shoot.

Ten-pound camera? Check.

Ten-pound tape deck? Check.

Five-pound tripod? Check.

Microphone and two, three-quarter-inch tapes, all the necessary cords? Check.

The drive to the facility felt short, and more than a little tense, knowing the kind of shoot it was going to be. When we arrived, Brent got his camera and tape deck out, and I carried in the tripod.

"Good morning, Ms. Casas; the room is ready. There's a pink gown inside; please leave the opening to the front," said the receptionist.

"Good morning," I responded as she led me and Brent inside the small room with the massive mammogram machine.

"Brent, I'm going to step out of the room to change while you set up," I said. I had never had a mammogram before, and Brent had never done a story like this, either. It was something new for both of us.

"We are Mammo virgins!" I told Brent, attempting to lighten the moment. He smiled nervously, mirroring my own anxiety. I went into the room next door and quickly removed my top and bra and left on the skirt. I left the opening to the cotton gown in the front and wrapped it around my chest. I had never really liked my large breasts, or my body. I slowly turned the knob to the exam room and walked inside.

"This is so awkward Brent, please be careful how you shoot this, and pretend you didn't see anything," I said jokingly. The walls of the room were a light pink with a few pieces of artwork; it was decorated to make the stark room more welcoming.

Brent placed the camera at just the right angle toward the mammogram machine.

"Good morning, Ms. Casas. I'm Rosie, and I will be doing your baseline mammogram. Are you ready?" the technician asked me, with perfect professional but friendly detachment.

"As ready as I can be with a man pointing a camera at my breasts," I responded in a near whisper as the three of us tried to get past the awkwardness of the moment with humor.

Rosie grabbed my (DD) right breast with her two hands and plopped it on the cold plate. She was careful to not fully expose it, which I appreciated. Yet, my journalist's mind kept thinking, *How do I tell an important story about breast health without showing the actual breast?* Then I thought to myself, *I will do it very discreetly.*

I was horrified then, as she positioned my breast and squeezed it, flattening it into a pancake shape in between the two plates. I stood paralyzed as she got into position, saying, "Hold your breath, hold it, hold it. You can breathe now."

As the plates released my breast, and Brent got the perfect video and natural sound of the machine, I exhaled, tears rolling down my face. I wasn't crying because it hurt. I cried out of embarrassment that a coworker, and soon all of our KVIA-TV viewers, were going to see my bare breasts. I was sobbing, trying to regain my composure, when she came over to position me on the other side, plopping my left breast on the machine.

"Hold your breath sweetie, hold it, hold it, breathe. And you're done. You can get dressed," Rosie said with a smile.

I looked over at Brent, who seemed to be having trouble looking into my eyes. He, too, was embarrassed as I walked out of the room.

In the changing room, I shook, fumbling with my buttons, as I wiped the tears and pulled myself together. Our job wasn't done. We still had to shoot more video and interview the doctor on the importance of mammography before heading back to the station.

Awkward silence enveloped us both as we drove back to the station; the rawness and boldness of the story made us quiet and distant. Struggling with the need to break that tension, I said, "I'm sorry, Brent. It was a tough shoot, but it will have an impact on women who are afraid of getting a mammogram because they think it's too painful. It's for the greater good."

Brent smiled nervously and nodded in agreement. We arrived at the station, where I began checking the video, channeling my discomfort into crafting the story. The message was to let women know that early detection saves lives. Exposing my breasts could give women the courage to check theirs.

Brent and I worked together a few more years before he left KVIA for a job as Operations Manager at KFOX. When Brent learned about this chapter, he sent me this quote: "I thought your decision to demonstrate the importance of having a mammogram in a real, transparent, and vulnerable manner, took a lot of courage on your part. I was proud to be a part of this (your) story. Especially your concern for many Hispanic women and wanting to help break old taboos they often associate with this exam."

Year after year following that first mammogram, I made the trip to the imaging center, minus Brent. When I was diagnosed and learned that I would be losing both breasts, I thought back on that fateful day. I decided to share my journey on TV, digging deep and developing courage and strength in the person and body I disliked. I discovered that by accepting myself, and accepting the reality that I was going to lose my hair, lose my breasts, and possibly lose my life, that I was beautiful.

I knew I was beautiful inside and out, despite the hardships that lay ahead. For once, I was beginning to feel miraculously made. I kept questioning the paradox: *How is it possible that knowing that I'm going to be losing a part of me actually makes me feel whole?*

I couldn't answer that question, but one thing I know for sure, is that I emptied my mind and heart of all the negativity in my life, anchored firmly to my faith, opened my heart and mind, and realized my breasts are just a small part of who I am. They don't define me.

It took a cancer diagnosis for me to accept that I am so much more than my individual parts. I realized that my brokenness is beautiful because putting those pieces back together has yielded a woman who is whole, who is worthy. I am enough, enough to love myself. I am enough to be loved, and I feel like the woman God intended me to be. I am a woman of value. I am a woman of faith. I am embracing my vulnerabilities and flaws. In my brokenness, I have become more kind, compassionate, and grateful. I thank God every day for my health and the health of those I love; and I pray for grace for strangers who are fighting their own monsters.

The sunrises and sunsets I see each precious day are breathtaking because I see God in them. I am in awe of the beauty around me, especially the beauty inside people.

There is so much ugliness in the world, but even in that ugliness, there's beauty. I choose to find it, so I can celebrate and honor it. I am alive, and like you, a work in progress. I found my true voice. I love with passion. I live with purpose. I am enough. I am beautiful.

CHAPTER TWO

God-Incidence

"When was the last time you had a tetanus shot?" she asked casually.

Lying half-naked on an exam table following a pap smear, I couldn't think of an answer to her question. My physician, Dr. Georgina Escandon, had known me a long time, but (like many of you, probably) I had a hard time looking at the person who'd just seen and looked inside the most intimate part of my body!

I responded, "I can't recall. Maybe when I was in college, about thirty years ago!"

Dr. Escandon chuckled. "I think you should get one," she suggested as she asked me to get dressed and walked out the door.

I had gone in for a checkup because I had been losing weight and was running low on thyroid meds. I've always tried to be on top of my health, and to know my body pretty well. I always make sure to get regular pap smears, mammograms, and blood work done to check on my cholesterol and blood glucose levels. In fact, I was the one who found the four-centimeter lump on my neck in 2010.

Minutes before the 10:00 p.m. newscast, I was in front of the bathroom mirror applying makeup. As my fingers moved toward the middle of my neck (TV makeup must be thorough!), right below the Adam's apple, I felt a lump the size of a walnut. It was round and felt spongy. I kept looking at it and moving it around, hoping it was just my imagination.

I rushed onto the set and told my coworkers what I had discovered. When we went to a commercial break, I asked them to touch it. My coanchor, Rick Cabrera, agreed there was something here. He felt something. I wasn't going crazy or imagining things.

In between stories, when it was time for Rick to read, I texted my cousin Lety, a registered nurse and breast cancer fighter, who gave me some names and numbers for doctors I could consult.

Six months and two surgeries later, I was diagnosed with follicular carcinoma, the second most common type of thyroid cancer. There are four types of thyroid cancer: papillary (is the most common), follicular, medullary, and anaplastic. The last two cancer types are more aggressive and difficult to treat. I was told, "If you have to have cancer, that's the cancer to get." I thought it was the end of the world, but I later found out they were right. For most people, thyroid cancer is manageable.

Back in Dr. Escandon's office, I agreed to the tetanus shot. A swab on the arm, a needle stick, and it was done. In short order, I was dressed and leaving the office with a six-month prescription for Synthroid, orders for blood work, a mammogram scheduled for four months later, and a clean bill of health. Despite the big red bump on my arm, my blood pressure and vitals were good, and I'd get results from the pap smear later that week.

The weight loss I had been concerned about was explained by changes in behavior. I was exercising four to five days a week and making better food choices. Lactose intolerance got me to eliminate ice cream, milk, and cheese from my diet. Even now, I eat very little bread unless it's flourless, or it's fresh out of the oven at a restaurant. I like a thick medium steak once in a while but eat mostly chicken, fish, and vegetables. I was taking cha-cha, salsa, and tango lessons at a nearby ballroom, and the lessons sometimes replaced dinner, so naturally, I was going to slim down!

Later that evening, I began suffering flu-like symptoms. I went home for dinner and chose a nap instead. My body felt achy, my energy zapped. I went to my bedroom, got under the covers (trying not to ruin my TV makeup since I had to go back to the station later that night) and fell right to sleep. Thirty minutes later, I woke up groggy, popped an ibuprofen, touched up my makeup, and headed back to work. I was so tired, I barely got through the newscast. Counting the minutes until the newscast ended, I just wanted to be home and in bed.

Days later, the flu-like symptoms went away, but the pain and swelling wouldn't. The bump on my arm actually got bigger, but I was too excited and distracted to think about it. I'd invested a lot of time and money into a planned trip with friends to New York City and Washington DC, and I wasn't going to let that once-in-a-lifetime trip get sidelined because of a reaction to a tetanus shot! I was tougher than *that*; although every time I put something in my suitcase, I felt the bump.

With suitcases and bags in hand, our considerable crew—friends Nicole Grado, who is also a thyroid cancer survivor and Toni Sides along with our kids—hopped on the plane headed to the Big Apple. Nicole and I had met when I announced on KVIA I had thyroid cancer. She showed up at the station with bags of sour candy. "You need to suck on the sour candy to help stimulate the salivary glands during the radioactive iodine treatment," she said when she handed me the bags of Sour Punch and Sweet Tarts. Although Nicole is 20 years younger than me, we made a special connection and developed a lifelong friendship. Toni and I had met a few years before and had many things in common. We have adult children and were healing from separation and divorce. We took dance lessons together!

Our hopes for a magical adventure were fulfilled. Once in New York, we met up with another friend, Sandra Terrazas, making us a group of eight. Sandra was also a new friend. Toni introduced us when my son Marcos was looking for a college internship. He was studying Exercise Science at Truman State University and needed a summer program. Sandra is a physical therapist and owner of Spectrum Therapy Consultants with clinics throughout El Paso. It was a spring afternoon, with salmon and kale salads at G2 Geogeske's on North Stanton, when we formed a special bond and began a friendship. Marcos gained a summer internship but with Sandra in our lives we gained so much more. The Gang of eight set out to conquer the Big Apple. We took a boat ride near the Statue of Liberty, went salsa dancing, visited Times Square, saw a Broadway musical, laughed with controversial comedian Dave Chappelle, and rode bikes in Central Park. We had delicious meals, went shopping, and snapped pictures at Rockefeller Plaza as dozens of people ice-skated in the rink below.

Life was good!

Sandra, who is also a physical therapist, hadn't planned to continue to DC with us, but after some prodding and persuading at a farmer's market in Manhattan, she changed her mind. I'm eternally thankful that she did.

The following day, we boarded the train to DC, ready for whatever adventures awaited us! The ride was fun, as we traded stories and plans for the future. I was newly divorced and dating, my work life was satisfying, my children were healthy, and I had enough Synthroid to last the next six months. Life couldn't be more perfect!

We stayed at the Watergate Hotel and spent the first evening enjoying cocktails and expensive pizza on the top patio. The fire pits were on to help keep us warm in the crisp air and the light breeze coming off the Potomac River. An illuminated Capitol building in the distance filled our eyes. It was a magical night.

The following morning, we were scheduled to get a tour of the White House and Capitol Hill. I had made arrangements through

El Paso congressman Beto O'Rourke's office for a behind-the-scenes tour. We got up early, took turns using the shower, and planned for another busy day.

After my shower, I stood in front of the steamed-up mirror to wipe it down. As I started to put on my bra, I noticed something strange on the inside of my arm. A long vein was protruding, extending down from my armpit to the inside of my elbow. It was on the other side of the bump caused by the tetanus shot administered ten days before. It stopped me in my tracks. I hadn't noticed it before. I called out to Sandra to show her.

She pulled me out of the bathroom and sat me on a chair. She extended my arm. As I was about to show her, she said, "I see it. You have a cord and two lymph nodes."

A cord and two lymph nodes?

I asked, "What is it? . . . Should I be worried?"

Her face showed her concern. Sandra didn't like what she saw.

"Who's your oncologist?" she quickly asked. "You need to see him as soon as we get back."

"Dr. Valilis?" I asked.

Sandra replied, "Yes, you have a cord and swollen lymph nodules at the end. Women with breast cancer develop this type of swelling."

I sat quietly, trying to take in what Sandra had just told me. My heart sank, and I felt a knot in my stomach. I told myself over and over that it wasn't breast cancer. I had to remain positive. After all, things were going so well in my life; she couldn't be right. Life was good. My family and I had already been through so much the last eighteen months. We deserved to be happy and at peace. Separation and divorce after thirty-two years of marriage may have broken us, but we had moved forward, rebuilt our connections, and I had even found love again. My heart and mind roiled with emotions.

I put that information away and finished getting ready for our tour of Capitol Hill. We grabbed a quick bite for breakfast, called an Uber, and headed out. We were treated to a special tour through the back halls and offices. We learned lots of information about the history of paintings and spaces in the Capitol building. We snapped many pictures, asked many questions, and left proud of our American history.

On our way back to the hotel, we spotted a small Catholic church. A family tradition, we went in, lit a candle, and offered a prayer for a safe flight home. I thanked God for keeping us safe in New York City and Washington, DC, and I asked Him for good health. I knelt down in one of the pews and prayed Sandra's assessment was wrong. I prayed that whatever was on my arm was a reaction from the tetanus shot. In the middle of my prayer, I also remembered a phrase my brother used when my mother was dying of congestive heart failure and repeated it several times:

"God help me to accept Your will and do Your will."

My heart was open to receive what lay ahead. I hoped it would be just another scare.

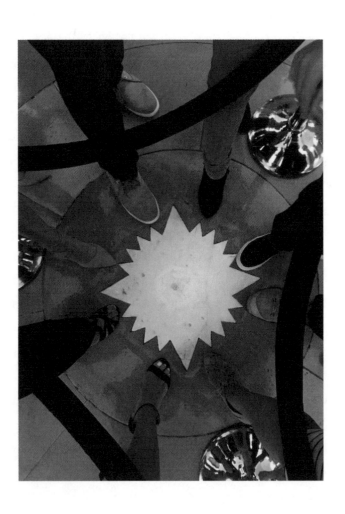

CHAPTER THREE

No Puede Ser!

Denial.

It has to be the tetanus shot.

Snap another picture.

It couldn't be cancer.

Smile!

It couldn't be breast cancer.

This is one of my favorite pictures from that trip:

Each of us with our right foot surrounding a star with four large points and sixteen small ones on the floor inside the Capitol Building. It's a compass star, which is actually a grid of how the streets in Washington are laid out and numbered. The picture is poignant to me, not only because it brought all eight of us together, but also because it symbolized an invisible grid of the twists and turns that would mark the journey ahead—a truth I couldn't yet face. As my mind flooded with thoughts of denial, we headed back home to El Paso.

The morning after our return, at 9:00 a.m. sharp, I called my oncologist, Dr. Panagiotis Valilis. He was available that afternoon, but I wasn't. I had a date with my BMAC (beloved monogamous adult companion), and I wasn't going to miss it!

Yes, I know . . . priorities!

Jimmy and I were three months into our relationship, and we hadn't seen each other in ten days. I admit, love clouded my judgment. It always does. Too enamored to take time out to take care of my health, I couldn't wait to see him and tell him all about the trip. We met for dinner.

We sat in the restaurant and held hands as I gave Jimmy every last detail, and he smiled and listened. I was tired, but wired, and talking fast. I get that way when I'm nervous. He stole a few kisses in between, as I told him about the Broadway musical we saw and the night we got caught in the rain leaving the dance club. Even though he's visited New York City many times, he listened intently as I described our bike ride in Central Park and the comedian whose politically incorrect jokes we laughed at, seeing it all through my eyes. His own eyes flashed with delight as I related, in detail, our private tour of Capitol Hill and shared all the pictures, including a night at Yankee Stadium, watching the Yankees play the Boston Red Sox, and the wedding we witnessed atop a building on Wall Street, and how the four of us adults shared a bottle of expensive champagne.

Jimmy's face lit up as I remembered how we rocked a boat on the Hudson as we danced to "Despacito," one of my favorite songs. He remembered we had danced to that same song on the 11th-floor balcony of the condominium he was living in when we first met.

I deliberately didn't tell Jimmy about the one thing that almost ruined our trip. I didn't feel it was the right time to show or tell him about the cord on my arm, or the sobering words Sandra spoke in the hotel room.

We enjoyed a beautiful evening together. We made memories and continued to build a special bond between us, having found love again later in life. At that moment, that was all that mattered.

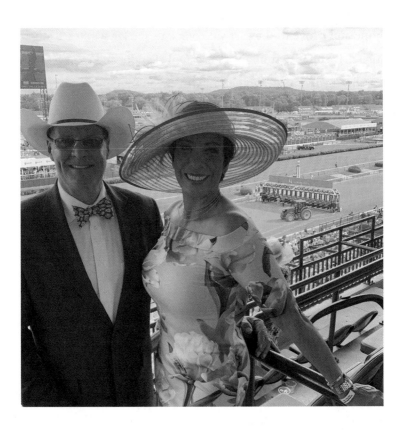

Getting the opportunity to get to know someone at that level is a privilege. I felt special. I had almost forgotten how it felt to be alive, but with Jimmy, I was moving on with my life. I was in a happy place and couldn't imagine leaving it. I felt like a seventeen-year-old who had a crush on the captain of the football team, or in the case of a choir girl like me, the president of the Choir Club! I didn't have a care in the world, and I wanted to stay in that space as long as possible. Love is a wonderful feeling. It would be that love interest and positivity that would get me through the dark days, weeks, and months to follow.

Friday morning, I got into my car filled with courage and hope and drove to the east side office to see Dr. Valilis. It was a long drive on I-10 from my house. Only Sandra and I knew of the appointment. I wasn't going to alarm anyone about the visit to the cancer center until I had concrete information.

I left the house early to avoid heavy traffic. I drove past the University of Texas-El Paso, admiring the Bhutanese architectural buildings of my alma mater. I recalled the twenty-five years it took me to earn my broadcast journalism degree. I definitely had endurance going for me!

To the right of I-10 is Mexico, with just a mesh fence and the Rio Grande dividing the two countries. The river didn't have much water running through it, months after the annual release from the Elephant Butte Reservoir that brings much-needed water to area farmers for irrigation.

The differences between the US and Mexico sides at that point of the border are stark. Gorgeous architecture on one side, and a shanty town of corrugated metal homes on the other. As I do every time I drive past, I noticed the differences and thanked God I was on the US side, where the likelihood of dreams coming true with hard work and dedication is much higher.

Lost in those thoughts, I didn't realize I was going about eighty miles an hour. Negotiating a curve going eighty probably wasn't a very good idea, and I slowed down. I had zoomed past a lot of cars, and the world around me seemed as if it were moving in slow motion. So many questions before me, my eyes filled with water, but I didn't let any tears fall. Over and over, I reminded myself that I had to be strong. I could not get ahead of myself and let worry or fear take over.

I finally saw the sign off the freeway: Texas Oncology. I pulled into the parking lot in front of the burnt orange building. I spotted Sandra getting out of her car and walking toward me. She was wearing tennis shoes and scrubs, so she could head into the office directly after the appointment. She had a forced smile, and I picked up on her vibe. I read her eyes behind her sunglasses. They weren't bright, like when she's happy. Still, they gave me hope, as did Sandra's reassuring hug. As the glass doors to the cancer center opened, we knew deep inside that my life, and the lives of those I love, were about to change forever.

"Good morning, Ms. Casas. You can go right in. Dr. Valilis will be with you shortly," said the friendly receptionist.

I walked a little ahead of Sandra. I could hear her heavy breathing, and I felt concern in her footsteps. The nurse took my temperature and blood pressure and asked me to change into a gown before Dr. Valilis entered the room. Moments later, I heard the knock on the door, and he walked in with his crisp white doctor's robe, a warm smile, and red cheeks. And then the questions started as he touched the bump on my arm from the tetanus shot. Did my arm hurt? It felt hot and tender. He looked at my underarm and noticed the cord and swollen lymph nodes; then he asked how long had it been there. He examined my breasts with light palpations.

Closing my paper exam gown, he said, "Infections after a vaccine are common. The site probably got infected, so I am prescribing an antibiotic. I would also like you to get an ultrasound of the bump on your arm, and while you're there, have them check both breasts and lymph nodes, as a precaution."

"Just a precaution?" I asked, my tone seeking reassurance.

Dr. Valilis answered, "Yes," with his signature smile and beautiful Greek accent.

Sandra and I looked at each other and raised our eyebrows. I got dressed and walked out with a prescription for antibiotics and an order for an ultrasound seven days away. Sandra and I hugged, and I thanked her again for her support and care.

I don't know what she was thinking as she left for work, but I kept thinking she may have been wrong about the cord in my arm. I was on top of my health. I'd had a mammogram eight months before and got the "all clear." For years, doctors had been keeping an eye on some areas of my breasts. I had several cysts aspirated over the years and a few painful needle biopsies. Surprisingly, I wasn't overly concerned. I was too busy living, I told myself, to stop and imagine that anything was wrong.

All I knew at the moment was that I had to drop off the prescription, complete 7 days of antibiotics, and have an ultrasound on Saturday, August 26th, the day my older brother Fernando was coming to visit from Portland.

I began my seven-day regimen of antibiotics and started planning for his arrival. The week went by quickly, with the everyday challenges at home and at work. Having two sons at home is a daily adventure.

Saturday arrived as I took the last pill, and I headed to my ultrasound appointment. I wouldn't need the order for the mammogram Dr. Escandon wrote up for December; instead, I would be getting a more thorough exam of both breasts, lymph nodes, and the bump on my arm.

"Good morning, Ms. Casas," said the receptionist at Diagnostic Outpatient Imaging.

I have a long medical history there, dating back several years. "Good morning," I responded with a smile.

"Please go in through that door and follow the nurse," she said as she pointed the way.

I was quickly taken to the ultrasound room, where I was asked to remove my blouse and bra, put on a gown, and climb on the examining table. I laid down and covered myself. The room felt warm and comfortable. I was texting. I had a busy and exciting day planned for my brother's visit.

The technician flipped off the light switch, pulled the curtain, and sat in her chair to work the machine. "How are you this morning?" she asked.

"I'm here, and I hope the results turn out okay," I answered.

"Let's take a look," she said as she dabbed some gel on my right breast and began gliding the wand over it.

I put my phone away, closed my eyes, and began going over plans for the day in my head. Every time I opened my eyes, she kept stopping and typing. It felt like an unusually long exam. I couldn't look over at the screen, and the room was too dark to observe her expression. I distracted myself, mapping out my day while she was mapping out my breasts.

It wouldn't be the first time my breasts sent out an alarm for a follow up, but I didn't have time, didn't want to make time to imagine the possibilities. My head was spinning with a list of things to do that morning.

As my mind spun, the ultrasound technician finished going over both breasts, armpits, and right arm.

"We're done. You can get dressed now," she said as she handed me a towel to wipe the gel off my breasts. She added, "I'll make sure the radiologist sees the films and shares the results stat."

I didn't like hearing that word. I had always been escorted to the radiologist's office, where Dr. Bushka read it in front of me. I would get the written results later in the mail. I tried not to find it unusual.

I smiled as I buttoned my blouse, and said, "Thank you." I went about my day without a care in the world. I was on a mission to play host to my brother, who was a couple of hours away from landing.

That afternoon, when my brother arrived, the fun started. Fernando is fourteen years older than me. He makes me laugh. He also really enjoys my chile-con-queso. I prepared a pan full of Hatch green chile with thinly sliced onions and small chunks of tomato. The cheese goes on top and melts slowly under the lid. We sat at the kitchen counter, and he proceeded to make bite-size taquitos. More than a dozen tortillas later, he had finished the entire pan of chile!

I cleaned up the kitchen, threw the plates in the dishwasher, and got ready for the baseball game and concert. Fernando is well-traveled, and he's been to famous baseball stadiums, but I wanted to show him our beautiful Southwest University Park, home of the El Paso Chihuahuas. El Paso City Hall was imploded to make room for the $72 million stadium in the downtown area, and if you get to sit in a strategic area, you can see the famous Star on the Mountain.

It is 459 feet long, 278 feet wide, and has 459 light bulbs. It's been up in its current dimensions since 1946. It used to be that the bulbs were switched on only in December. The "Star on the Mountain" became an El Paso tradition during the Christmas season.

In 1980, the Star remained lit for 444 days during the Iran hostage crisis. In 1990, during the Gulf War, the Star once again remained lit for a year in support of Fort Bliss and all US troops stationed with Operation Desert Storm.

Now it shines brightly every night. It's dedicated to the residents of El Paso, but an individual or organization can pay to have it lit in their honor. For me, it's more than just a pretty star with white bulbs. It is my guiding light when I find myself lost. I look toward the mountain, and when I see the star, I know I'm home.

It was a clear evening as Fernando and I arrived at the ballpark. We both sat in awe of the breathtaking view of the beautiful ballpark with the star in the backdrop.

We settled into our seats and watched a few plays. We socialized, took selfies, made new friends, and exchanged jokes with old ones. Fernando and I walked a couple of blocks to the Plaza Theater for the concert. He had been at the Plaza Theater when he was a teenager, but he had not been back in several decades. Fernando hadn't seen the $38 million renovation. The Plaza Theater now hosts concerts and Broadway musicals. Inside, it's stunning, with a starlit ceiling, balconies, and red velvet seats. We walked into the sold-out concert and made our way to the first row.

The musicians began taking their spots and tuning their instruments. The sounds of violins, guitars, trumpets, and piano filled the theater. The excitement started to build. And then the music started, and singer Shaila Dúrcal walked on stage with a colorful long dress and filled the theater with her sultry voice. I knew all the songs she sang, songs I sang when I dreamed of being a singer. The lyrics reminded me about the past—the good, and the not so good, times. I sang along and laughed at the jokes, and I cried at some of the lyrics. It was a gorgeous evening, all the more precious with my brother and dear friends around me. We walked across the street to the Camino Real Hotel, another building steeped in rich history. We enjoyed a few glasses of wine at the Dome Bar just below the beautiful stained glass dome above the bar. We toasted to old songs and new friends. We toasted to life.

Sunday morning, I drove Fernando to meet his longtime friends for a golf trip to Ruidoso, New Mexico. He and his friends from Jefferson High School get together to play golf at a different destination every year. As luck would have it, that year it was just three hours from El Paso, where I live.

Right place. Wrong time?

No.

Right place. Right time.

I got out of the car and said hello to Fernando's friend and one of the wives. Her head was wrapped in a scarf. She was bald, frail, and pale. Chemo had taken her hair in her fight against stomach cancer. We chatted for a little while, and we both raved about our oncologist, Dr. Valilis.

I recall looking at her and realizing that she reminded me of the frailty of life and how cancer changes people. I noticed her gray skin and sad, sunken eyes. I gave her a hug and wished her luck on her journey.

As fate would have it, in a matter of weeks, I would be embarking on the same journey with the same uncertainty.

I waved goodbye to the group of friends and said to Fernando: "Have a great time. Love you too much, see you Wednesday."

CHAPTER FOUR

Moment of Truth

Monday morning, 6:45 a.m.

My alarm shrieked me awake, letting me know it was time to get Andres up, make his breakfast, and get him to school. He was in 8th grade at Hornedo Middle School, and we liked to leave early and get there before traffic got heavy. The start of *his* day didn't mean *I* had to be "camera ready," so I threw on a baseball cap and slipped on some tennis shoes, shorts, and a workout shirt.

Mondays meant I could either take a spin class or shake my groove thing at Zumba. Because I'd overindulged during my fantastic weekend with friends and family, I chose the biking class so I could burn more calories. I'd had too much food, and too much wine, but could never get enough laughter. When my heart is filled with love and joy, I laugh harder—the kind of laugh that comes from deep inside. The weekend had given me a lot of those.

After dropping off Andres, I realized I had forgotten my cycling shoes, so I stopped by my house to get them. Shoes in hand, I headed to the garage. Just then, my phone rang, Dr. Valilis' name flashing on the screen.

"Good morning, Dr. Valilis," I said, concern under my breath.

"Good morning, Estela! I got the results back from the radiologist, and you need three biopsies," he declared in his cool, professional tone.

I froze at his words. My tennis shoes felt stuck to the wooden floors. I couldn't move.

Breathlessly, I asked, "Biopsies. How many?"

He answered efficiently, "Three. One on each breast and a lymph node under the right armpit have to be checked. The lump on your arm is of no concern."

"Okay, thank you, doctor. I'll call Dr. Landeros to set up an appointment," I answered softly, trying to keep the tremor in my voice under control.

I had heard him clearly, but it took more time for me to understand the information he'd shared. My knees buckled. I felt I might faint; blood was rushing to my head. My thoughts went into overdrive as I attempted to catch my breath. Alone in the middle of my dark bedroom, sitting on my unmade bed, there was no one to hold me and tell me everything was going to be okay. With tears rolling down my face, I slipped down to my knees and began praying.

"Please God, help me get through this. Let me accept Your will and do Your will."

I kept repeating that phrase over and over, and I included the

Lord's Prayer and a couple of Hail Marys. In my anguish, I thought the more I prayed, the faster God might hear my plea.

But I like solutions, action. I got up, trying to figure out what I was going to do next.

Who do I tell first?

How do I tell my children?

I answered my own questions.

Don't say anything until you get the results back from the biopsies.

Don't get ahead of yourself and jump to conclusions.

I calmed myself down by taking long, deep breaths. I tried to meditate and be more conscious of my breaths. Suddenly, my mind started wandering . . .

Strapped in the seat of a roller coaster, I see myself alone and making a steep climb to the top, with a bird's-eye view of the city lights. I begin hyperventilating, knowing I'll soon be zooming down the rails toward a big drop. (I get nauseated on roller coasters, so I'm not a big fan.) *But instead of panicking, I take a deep breath and let myself go to enjoy the ride. There is no other way to get through the terrifying minutes, other than to just let go of the rail that secured me in the seat, raise both arms, and let the wind hit my face. The roller coaster comes to a slow stop at the bottom. I unbuckle myself because there is no attendant, get off, and don't look back.*

Focusing back into the moment, I realized my vision was a metaphor for the coming challenges. This journey would be like a roller coaster ride, with its ups and downs and sharp curves. I realized that I was going to experience moments that could be terrifying and take my breath away, and there would be moments to let go, embrace the journey, and lean on God.

As I said, I like solutions and action, so I called my trusted surgical oncologist, Dr. Mark Landeros. Eight years earlier, he was the surgeon who successfully removed my thyroid. He had also treated me for previous issues in my breasts.

"Hi, Dr. Landeros. I got an ultrasound Saturday, and Dr. Valilis says I need three biopsies. When can you see me?" I asked, all business, all action.

"Come in tomorrow afternoon," he answered.

So fast. It was all happening so fast, and yet, my conversation with Sandra in that hotel room seemed far, far away—like it was a different me . . . a lifetime ago.

Needing to clear my thoughts, I jumped in the shower. Water fell from the showerhead, and from my eyes. I sobbed, blaming myself for not having caught it earlier. I threw a litany of accusals at myself:

I didn't eat enough vegetables.

I should have eaten more salmon and fish for the omega-3s. I shouldn't have eaten the dark chocolate I'd read was good for my heart.

With so many questions and emotions running through me, I turned toward the shower head and let the water hit my face and breasts. Salty tears merged with the warm water down my chest, stomach, legs, and feet until they swirled down the drain. I wasn't angry. I was sad and disappointed. I felt I didn't have anyone to blame but myself.

I deliberately looked down at my breasts. We'd been through a lot together. I was an early bloomer. When I was ten years old,

I got my period and developed big breasts, which had caused me embarrassment as a child, and sometimes pain as an adult. Thankfully, I'd been able to have a reduction done, and without judgment or resentment, they had still filled with milk to nurse my three children. They had served me well, but now they were making me sick. Instead of giving life, as they had for Carolina, Marcos, and Andres, they might be killing me.

I got out of the shower, wrapped myself in a towel, and crawled back into the still unmade bed. I hugged a pillow tightly and found myself in a fetal position, sobbing.

I knew.

I knew the biopsies would turn up something bad.

I knew I was in for the fight of—and for—my life.

I also knew, as tough and as painful as it was, action was my way through. I forced myself out of bed and got ready for work. I slipped on a dress and heels, and applied some makeup, which served as my armor against the emotions coming at me like waves on a moody sea.

I told myself I had to leave the house acting like there was nothing wrong in my life. No one could know what was really happening inside my heart and head and growing inside my chest. I was terrified, but I was also determined that no one would know my secret . . . yet.

I pulled into the KVIA parking lot and got out of the car, holding my makeup bag in one hand and my purse in the other, smiling. I smiled at everyone in the hall as I made my way to the newsroom. I flashed that forced smile to my colleagues, and said, "Hello everyone," making my way into my office, my momentary sanctuary. I sat there for a few seconds, relaxing my forced smile, before going into the editorial meeting. I wondered how I was going to put it back on and hold myself together.

As I gathered my thoughts, plotting my meeting survival strategy, my phone started vibrating.

"Ms. Casas, this is Alicia from Dr. Landeros's office. Can you come in tomorrow morning at 9:00? The doctor needs to do the biopsies."

Morning? I thought he'd scheduled an afternoon appointment. Why the rush?

"Of course," I answered, fighting for composure. "Thank you."

I hung up and broke down at my desk, knowing my determination to keep my secret was slipping away. I didn't want anyone to see me sobbing, so I gathered my things and walked out. Later, I called KVIA's General Manager Kevin Lovell, explained why I left and asked for the rest of the week off.

My journey had begun, for real.

I was about to become a statistic: the one in eight women diagnosed with breast cancer.

I thought I knew, after telling the stories of other "one in eight" women; I thought I understood their journeys.

I had no idea.

CHAPTER FIVE

Fear Fiesta

Facing a cancer diagnosis incites fear.

If you've come this far on the journey with me, you know the fear, at first, was of the unknown. There is still a lot more of the journey to come, but first, I want to talk about the fear, the consistent companion on a journey like this one.

It's a much bigger fear than the kind that comes from knowing you're about to get a "cintarazo" or belt whipping from Dad, or the so called "chancla" or slipper flung perfectly at your head by a disappointed Mom. (My mother never did that, but I heard of others who did!)

No, this fear was something else—something at once both familiar and new.

One time, it rushed over my body like a wave. The hurt and desperation traveled from my toes to the top of my head and found the soft spot in my broken heart. Until then, I hadn't realized a heart could break like that from something other than lost love.

It's the kind of fear that makes your eyes swell with tears and twists your insides into knots deep inside your body. It's fear of the unknown, and it's the fear of facing the real and raw possibility of hearing, "There's nothing else we can do. You have weeks to live."

It's the fear of learning my time with my children, family, and friends could soon be up. It's the disappointment of knowing I might not be enjoying a glass of red wine, or the magic of a fiery red sunset in October. It's that fear that leaves me wondering whether I might die alone and worrying about the broken hearts and emptiness I would leave behind.

Fear is such a powerful emotion that if you let it take over, it will send you into a tailspin of depression; a deep, dark hole from which you may not be able to climb out.

But fear is also nearly inevitable, and we must give ourselves that grace sometimes. I've earned the right to feel sorry for myself. (And so have you.) I am the only one who can feel sorry for me. Just as you are the only one who can feel sorry for your own life.

I had several moments, especially early on in the fear of the unknown, when I caught myself falling into an abyss. Fortunately, the moments, agonizing and seemingly endless, were actually less than five minutes.

My dear Sandra told me I was allowed to have Fear Fiestas.

"Stell, they can't be longer than five minutes, but you better use that time wisely. You can let it all out in five minutes; and then you pull yourself together and straighten out," Sandra said the day we saw the doctor the first time.

So, I listened. I set a timer on my phone when I discovered that my emotions and fears were getting the best of me. With the rush of tears, my swirling head, and my heart and body shaking, I let it all out. I cried and cried, letting out the guttural sounds from my throat:

"Ahiiii Dios mío!"

I chose to have those moments when I was alone. I didn't want anyone to see me weak and vulnerable.

I've cried for different reasons throughout my life, as have you all, I imagine. Tears of joy after the birth of my three children. I've cried tears of sorrow following the death of my parents, knowing the people who loved me the most were gone forever. I've cried tears of disappointment after a failed marriage. I've cried tears of losing a friend to an untimely death.

My Fear Fiestas felt different. I was confronting my mortality. I've always known that we die every day we live. We never know if we'll have the privilege of opening our eyes the following morning. Now I faced the possibility of that happening sooner than I felt ready for.

My tears felt different. When you're confronted by a potentially fatal diagnosis, maybe the fluids in the body *do* react differently. Along with the saltiness, these tears had a taste of regret.

I started thinking that I should have been less prideful, less judgmental, and more understanding. I should have been a more loving mother and wife. I should have been a kinder daughter and sister. I should have been a more caring friend.

I should have traveled more extensively. I should have eaten more vegetables and sipped expensive wine. I should have taken up a sport. I should have learned to tango. I should have gotten a nose job and my toes separated. I should have flown with the Thunderbirds; I should have gone skydiving. I should have recorded an album. I should have bought a house with a view to enjoy sunrises and sunsets. I should have driven a red convertible to feel the sun and wind in my hair.

I should not have been so afraid to *love* more deeply and *live* more fully.

I had to decide not to let fear cheat me out of giving cancer a chance to transform me. I wouldn't let fear cheat me out of making me a better person. The Fear Fiestas allowed me to see that it was time to let God work in me and get me through. He would remove fear from my heart and head in time.

I never asked God, "Why me?" I asked Him to *show me* the answer. I asked Him to guide me, and for the strength and courage to face whatever He had planned for me. I asked Him to show me how to face my fears with grace and dignity. I felt I'd failed Him and really didn't feel I could ask Him to cure me. A cure would be a bonus!

I stole five minutes for my Fear Fiestas. But it is on His time, and He is the one who is allowing me to live life to the fullest, without regrets.

CHAPTER SIX

Topless and Terrified

Forced smiles and soft "good mornings" greeted my friend, Patti Aguayo Tieman, and me as we passed the nurses' station inside Dr. Mark Landeros's office. Patti had met me in the waiting area because she didn't want me to go it alone. She's detail-oriented and takes copious notes. Her background is also in journalism, and she always carries a large purse, with pens and paper.

"You'll probably forget everything you hear today, so I'll take notes. That way you'll look back and won't have to try to remember; it'll all be here." Patti smiled as she pointed to her notebook. I smiled because she made sense. It would all be on paper, documented without question.

Dr. Landeros's longtime nurse, Alicia, led us into the small exam room. It was dark and cold. I glanced at the surgical tray next to the exam table, covered in crisp white paper. It was located in the middle of the room, and it was propped up like a throne of reality, just waiting for me. (And me with no crown!) Next to it was an ultrasound machine. Everything looked ominous.

Before Dr. Landeros came in, Alicia asked me several questions as Patti jotted down my answers.

"Ms. Casas, please take off your bra and put on this gown with the opening in the front," Alicia instructed.

Embarrassment flooded me as I realized my longtime friend was about to see my bare breasts. Patti helped remove my bra and set it, and my blouse, on the chair she was sitting on. She smiled as if to say, "It's okay, I have breasts too."

I adjusted my gown, sat up straight, and visualized adjusting my crown. With no room for modesty, but plenty for imagination, I laughed silently to myself. Humor was my refuge.

The crackle of crinkled paper was the only thing breaking the silence of the room as everyone took their place on stage. Me on my throne, Patti in the corner chair, and Alicia next to the surgical tray. The minute felt choreographed, with strategic and precise movements as the performance was about to get underway.

Dr. Landeros walked in with his usual friendly disposition and gave me a hug.

"Hello, Estela. I've read over the report, and looked at the images Dr. Boushka sent over. Now we need to take some tissue and send it to the lab to find out what it is," he said matter-of-factly.

I responded jokingly, "We meet again under these unfortunate circumstances!"

I've known Dr. Landeros for several years. He's an excellent physician with a beautiful bedside manner, and he answers my phone calls. Every time.

Dr. Landeros grabbed a pair of pink gloves and proceeded to tell me, "It's going to hurt a little as I insert the instrument. I will leave a tiny clip inside to mark the site. You'll hear something that sounds like a stapler. I'll be using the ultrasound transducer to help me find the tumors. I'm sorry if I hurt you."

I heard him sorting through the surgical instruments, the sound amping up my anxiety. I didn't have the courage to watch him perform the biopsies.

"I'm going to get started now; you'll feel a needle prick. That's just to numb the area," he said softly.

He proceeded to apply gel on my right breast, and with the help of the ultrasound transducer, he searched for the tumor, which he quickly found. "Here it is," he said as tiny, jawed forceps dug in to bite samples of the tumor.

It hurt. The numbing meds just covered the surface. I felt the instrument piercing through my breast and into the tumor deep inside my chest. I kept staring at the ceiling, working through the pain with deep breaths. He saw me squirming.

"I'm so sorry. I need to get a good sample of the tissue," he said.

Tears escaped from the corners of my eyes as I said, "I'm okay, doctor; you do what you need to do."

I tried distracting myself by counting the small holes in the tiles above my head, but I couldn't. I kept flinching and had to start the count over and over again.

And Patti? She wasn't taking notes anymore. She was so terrified to see the procedure, she couldn't take her eyes away. I heard her gasping quietly as she shrank into the chair.

Dr. Landeros carefully removed the specimens from the right breast and placed the tissue inside a small glass tube. The tumor was a centimeter long and located at 11 o'clock, and it was four centimeters deep in my chest. He removed five fatty samples. Dr. Landeros got four specimens from the lymph node under the right armpit and deposited them in a second tube to send out to the pathology lab. All the poking, prodding, piercing, and digging sent bad vibes down my spine. I kept hearing a clipping sound, like a suction gun extracting the tissue. I prayed, telling myself to stay positive. Deep inside, I knew it wouldn't be good.

"On to the left side; are you doing okay?" Dr. Landeros asked.

I lied, and answered, "I'm okay."

The two-centimeter mass on the left side was located at ten o'clock. Dr. Landeros took four samples of the tumor and placed them in the third tube.

"We're all done. We'll send the samples to the lab, and Alicia will get you all cleaned up. We should have the results ready tomorrow," said Dr. Landeros as he took off his gloves and threw them in the trash before leaving the room.

I was shaking and still staring at the ceiling as Alicia used a tissue to wipe down my bloodied breasts. She carefully and quietly covered the biopsy sites with gauze and surgical tape that covered my entire breasts. As I got up, I noticed the blood-stained gauze and instruments in the sink. There were drops of blood that had dripped onto the white paper on the exam table.

Alicia handed me my bra and blouse, and she and Patti propped me up and helped me get dressed. I sat quietly, trying to calm myself and stop shaking.

I turned to look at Patti and she said, "Oh, Estela, you are incredibly brave and courageous." Alicia agreed, and I nodded my thanks; then we all walked out.

On the way to the front desk, I saw Dr. Landeros inputting information into the computer. I gently raised my bandaged arm to wave goodbye. The expression in his eyes told me he already knew what the lab would confirm. As a surgical oncologist, he knows what cancerous tissue looks like, and he had just extracted some cancerous tissue from my breasts.

We locked glances and exchanged tight smiles.

His smile told me, "I'm sorry."

Mine said, "Thank you."

"I'll call you with the results," he said.

He knew I knew the outcome. We both just needed a pathologist to confirm it on paper.

Patti and I walked to our cars and said goodbye.

"I truly appreciate you sharing your morning with me, and I'm sorry you had to see all that. I'll let you know when I hear back from Dr. Landeros," I said.

"Please keep me posted," Patti said, and headed to her car.

Even now, years later, I have no words to describe what passed between us that day. We've been friends for more than three decades, and certainly shared many special moments. But that morning, our shared vulnerability, pain, courage, and yes, fear, brought us closer than we had ever been.

It was a long drive back to the westside. I didn't cry. I couldn't cry. I had to redirect that energy to think, act, and pray.

The phrase I had been repeating, *"God help me to accept Your will and do Your will,"* expanded to include, *"God give me strength and courage to face whatever was ahead with grace and dignity."*

Jimmy had asked that I stop by and see him before I went into work, and I gladly honored that request. I went into his office, ready to hold it all together, and ended up breaking down in the middle of the executive suite. He stood up from his big leather chair and took me in his arms, and I cried. I unbuttoned my blouse and showed him my bandaged breasts. They had already started bruising. As his green eyes skimmed down my chest, I noticed his eyes welling up.

"You're going to be okay," he said as he rubbed my head.

We held each other tightly, trying to be positive and reassuring. We were going on a trip together in a week.

But we both knew the lab results were going to show cancer. We needed to know the type, stage, and grade.

Jimmy is a man of few words. When he's upset and hurting, he speaks even less, but his expression said it all. He felt sad and afraid for me. As he held me in his burly arms, nestled to his chest, I could hear his heart beating faster. He kissed my forehead and said, "Let me know as soon as you hear back from Dr. Landeros."

My breasts hurt, but my heart hurt more.

CHAPTER SEVEN

But I Floss Every Day...

I choose to have a good day, every day.

It's hard to wake up in a bad mood and have to put on a smile. I choose to wake up feeling blessed, happy, and ready to face the day with a positive attitude.

But the day after my biopsies, choosing the good day seemed unreachable. I couldn't muster enough energy. I hadn't slept well, but I didn't want to sleep. Exercise usually helped make me feel good, but I didn't feel like going to the gym. I wasn't hungry or tired or happy or sad. I was feeling anxious and out of sorts. My breasts were throbbing, I was restless, and I just didn't know what to do with myself.

I headed to the kitchen to make a cup of coffee. I added an

extra scoop, knowing I would need the extra caffeine to face the day. I stood in front of the coffee machine, nearly entranced, watching the brown water slowly drip into the carafe. The steady stream was soothing, so the ring of my cell phone startled me, even though I knew the call was coming.

"Good morning, Dr. Landeros!" I answered, with an enthusiasm I didn't feel.

"Good morning, Estela," he said in a low and deliberate voice that set off a warning in my body.

"I am so sorry, but you have invasive carcinoma in both breasts . . . bilateral breast cancer. The tumor on the right breast is more aggressive than the two-centimeter tumor on the left breast. The lymph node came back negative," he said.

I stood in silence in the middle of my kitchen, unable to will his voice to stop.

He continued.

"Your cancer is estrogen negative and progesterone negative. I am waiting for a third test, the FISH (fluorescence in situ hybridization) report, that takes a couple more days to complete. That will determine if you have HER 2 negative or positive cancer. We need to schedule you for a double mastectomy in two weeks."

I marveled at his ability to say things in one breath that actually stole mine and left me at a loss for words. I closed my eyes, trying to process what I had just heard on the other end of the phone.

"I have breast cancer?" I asked.

"Yes, you have cancer in both breasts, and we have to act quickly," he told me more urgently. "I have scheduled you for an

MRI at Total Care on the Westside tomorrow morning and a PET scan on Friday. We need to find out if the cancer has spread. Please come to my office on Friday. I am sorry."

My voice cracked as I replied, "Thank you. See you Friday."

"Dios mío!" I whispered as my knees buckled and my head started spinning. I found myself on one of the kitchen rugs, curled up in the fetal position. I began praying, with the sound of the coffee brewing like some kind of background hymn.

"God, give me the strength and courage to face this with grace and dignity. It's in Your hands. I can't do this alone."

And then the blame game started.

What did I do wrong? I reminded myself that I never missed a doctor or dental appointment. I flossed every day! I didn't eat dairy products, bread, tortillas, or pasta. Enchiladas, tacos, beans, or quesadillas were never on my plate. I was eating clean with fresh vegetables. Pork and processed meat aren't part of my diet, except for an occasional batch of huevos con chorizo. I was exercising and had dropped some weight. I'd had a mammogram just eight months earlier.

The blame game shifted to the guilt trip as the "should haves" came into my heart. I should have started sooner! I should have been more aware of my body! I should have spent more time with my children! I should have worked more to educate myself!

What happened?

I couldn't answer that question.

Shit happens.

Life happens.

I picked myself up off the floor and went to my bedroom,

stripped down to my underwear and got in front of the mirror to try to find the tumors growing in my chest. The cancer was deep; I could never have felt the tumors, even if I tried. I slowly, carefully removed the surgical tape and blood-tinged bandages, finding my breasts bruised from all the poking and prodding during the biopsies.

I suddenly felt *afraid of my own breasts.*

I didn't want to touch them, thinking I could activate the cancer and make it spread. I looked at my right breast, imagining the small tumor, slightly larger than the size of a pea. It was angry and more aggressive than the larger one in the left breast. A monster was growing inside my chest, and I'd had no clue. I had failed myself.

It was time to let my close circle know what was going on. The first person I called was my daughter in Dallas, who had just started a new job. The second person I shared the news with was Fernando, who was returning from the golf tournament in Ruidoso.

I spotted him as I turned the corner. There he was, standing in the front yard, suitcase and golf clubs by his side, and a trophy in his hand. I popped open the trunk, unlocked the door, and he got in the car. Fernando began describing the weekend in detail and how his friends made him laugh all day with their shenanigans. He was so happy and relaxed, the trophy resting in his lap.

He lifted it and said, "My name won't be engraved in this gold-plate. I came in second, and no one but you remembers second place! There's no prize money for second place, either."

I agreed, and we laughed.

I was only halfway listening to his conversation, too wrapped up in my world to pay close attention to what he was saying. Fernando's mouth kept moving, making words, but I couldn't understand. He asked, "Are you okay?"

I was so happy he asked, and I was thankful he had opened the door to share my emotions. He had no clue how my world had shifted in just three days.

I took a deep breath, held on tightly to the steering wheel, and while driving out of the neighborhood, said as directly as I could, "I have some bad news. On Monday, I got the results from the breast ultrasound, and on Tuesday, I had three biopsies. Dr. Landeros called yesterday with the news that I have bilateral breast cancer. I'm having an MRI in a couple of hours, and tomorrow, I'm scheduled for a PET Scan to determine if the cancer has spread. I will be having a double mastectomy on September 23rd. Can you come with me to those exams?"

The words had come out in a rush, spoken with my eyes on the road ahead. When I looked over at Fernando, his eyes were wide open and glassy. He sat quietly, and took his turn staring at the road, as if trying to comprehend what he'd just heard. His little sister, fourteen years his junior, who had survived divorce, and just found happiness again, was about to begin the fight of her life!

In typical big brother mode, he answered, "Absolutely, I'm here to help with anything you need."

Reassured for the moment, I didn't hesitate to go down the list of things to do.

"You can come with me to get the MRI today and PET scan tomorrow. Carolina gets in tonight. I haven't told the boys."

My sons Marcos and Andres didn't know anything yet. Marcos was working, and Andres was in school. I know God brought Fernando to El Paso to help us get through those tough first few days. Another God-Incidence. Nothing happens by chance.

With heavy, but hopeful hearts, Fernando and I walked into the Hospitals of Providence Women's center. We sat across from the pink wall dedicated to women fighting breast cancer. It's a mobile display called "Pretty in Pink," and the women are all dolled up. They all look strong and beautiful in pink dresses. Some had their bald heads wrapped in pretty pink scarves. Others wore wigs. The bravest posed bald. Some of the women were in remission; others were fighting, and others had lost their fight. I had seen the display before, but on that day, it felt even more sobering to me. They were all cancer sisters, and I was now one of them, as of the 1 in 300,000 women diagnosed each year.

Fernando and I sat in silence.

"Ms. Casas," said the nurse, turning to Fernando and adding, "She'll be back shortly."

She smiled and escorted me into another room with several dressing rooms. She asked me to change into a pink gown.

"I'll wait right here to take you to the exam room," she said.

I make small talk with most people I encounter, but I wasn't saying much that day. I had no words and nothing to say. She led me into the special room where the magnetic resonance imaging machine was located.

"Good morning," the technician greeted me.

I replied in kind as he helped me onto the massive machine. He began giving me instructions.

"I need to put an IV in your hand because your doctor ordered an MRI with gadolinium contrast. This exam will allow us to see three-dimensional images of your breasts and determine where the tumors are, and their size. You'll need to get on your tummy, place each breast in the compartments and lift your arms above your head. Here are some headphones to block out the sound. Can I find a special radio station you'd like to listen to?"

"I'd like to hear some classical music because it has no lyrics, so I can't sing along," I told him. He smiled.

My poor breasts had already been through so much. They had bruises to prove it! I was embarrassed by the fact that the technician saw them, but the shame went away quickly, knowing that results from that M-R-I could spell D-E-A-T-H.

In fact, as I thought about it, I realized I couldn't afford modesty anymore. After four days of having my breasts exposed and poked and prodded and handled and squished, I *couldn't* care who saw them. My breasts were no longer beautiful. By that point, they were ugly to me, and they were also making me sick. I wanted them gone, ripped out of my chest, thrown in a steel bowl, and (after the examination of the tissue under the microscope) incinerated!

The music started, helping to mitigate the tapping and thumping sounds of the massive machine. I prayed dozens of Hail Marys and Our Lord's Prayer in English and Spanish during the thirty-minute procedure. This meditation brought me comfort.

In between prayers, I felt as if I was in a combat zone, listening to the bullets flying past me, grazing my skin. I heard, "Don't move," over the intercom. I felt trapped. I thought, *This is the kind of thing that triggers PTSD*, post-traumatic stress disorder. I was getting a concentrated dose of trauma as I contemplated the future and the next steps in this journey.

Then I heard over the intercom, "Ms. Casas, we're all done. I'll be in to remove the IV so you can get dressed. Your results will be ready tomorrow."

I was dizzy and physically and emotionally exhausted. I moved unconsciously, making my way slowly back to the dressing room to change out of the gown and back into my clothes and high heels.

It was over, and I'd survived. Again. And I'd helped my doctors learn more about this ruthless disease, but it was still just the beginning.

I still had one of the toughest challenges before me: telling everyone else I loved that I had cancer.

CHAPTER EIGHT

When Like Turns to Amor!

As difficult as it was, I shared my cancer diagnosis with all of my immediate family.

I knew my three children were hurting and having to face the possibility of losing their mother. Both of my brothers and my sisters-in-law had been shocked to hear the news too. But I knew, despite the hurt and shock, that my family was there to support me through this. They were ready to join the fight with their unconditional love.

There was one person, though, whom I hadn't told.

Jimmy.

I was facing the devastating diagnosis, feeling responsible for inflicting pain on my family, and the possibility of losing my life.

I truly feared I was just a couple of hours away from losing a man who had come to mean a great deal to me.

We were really still getting to know each other. We'd met fourteen weeks earlier at St. Clair's winery in Mesilla, New Mexico. Toni, who brought Sandra into my life also brought Jimmy. The three of us met for brunch. Jimmy was wearing a blue plaid shirt, baseball cap, and brown Roapers. I noticed his deep dimples, green eyes, and friendly smile. He won over my attention when he said: "I'll have whatever wine she's having, she's the boss." After one glass of Malbec and friendly conversation we left and visited several wineries along Highway 28. We capped the night at Toni's house with more wine and dancing to Dwight Yoakam's "Guitars, Cadillacs." He showed me The Pretzel, the Spinout, and the Fall Down Dip.

Jimmy and I were going on our sixteenth date, *and* I was about to tell him I had cancer in both breasts and would have them removed three weeks later.

It was a lot to face emotionally in such a new relationship. Was it too much? I was afraid of being a burden on my children and my family. I feared losing my job and losing the new-found joy in my heart. What more could I lose? I was about to find out. I had been told many stories of men walking away from a relationship after learning their wife or girlfriend had developed cancer. I kept remembering a phrase a friend shared with me when her husband left her after doctors diagnosed her with cervical cancer: "When doctors remove your private parts, you are no longer a woman."

"Meet me at Pelican's. I want you to meet two friends of mine," Jimmy said over the phone.

"Okay," I responded. "I'd like you to meet my kids, and my

brother, who is here from Portland too. See you soon."

Jimmy wanted his friends to meet the new woman in his life. I wanted my family to meet the man who brought joy and companionship into my life too. I slipped on a nice dress and my signature high heels (*Familiar and comfortable . . . my armor of normalcy*) and headed to the restaurant.

I arrived at Pelican's to find Jimmy waiting for me at the door. I was struck anew with the thought of just how much I had grown to care for him. I took in his handsome face and his broad and strong chest, thinking how safe I felt there when he held me. I hoped that after this night, I would still find that to be true.

We greeted each other with bright smiles and three quick pecks on the lips.

(*Why is three the magic number? I like the number three because it's an odd number. One kiss is never enough; two kisses is okay, but three quick pecks is the perfect amount.*)

Jimmy grabbed my hand, and we walked into the dark bar. It was hopping.

Strangers asked me, "How are you?"

Inside, I felt like saying, "I'm not well." Instead, I said with a smile, "I'm good; how are you?"

I really didn't care how they were doing. I heard them speak, and I saw their lips moving, but I was too distraught to hear what they were saying. It was all a blur to my distracted mind.

The typical Friday night with happy hour drinks and live music wasn't normally my thing. I could never have the happy hour special, because I always had to go back to anchor the 10 p.m. newscast. That evening was an exception because I'd taken the day off, but it was hard to enjoy it, given my circumstances.

Everyone else was celebrating the end of the work week. "Great to see you!" someone said.

"Great seeing you too!" I answered automatically.

I focused hard on "keeping it together" long enough to get through it as I flashed friendly smiles, shook hands, and embraced acquaintances with quick hugs. The mingling and networking all felt so superficial and meaningless at that moment. I held on tightly to Jimmy's hand, but what I really needed was a hug, wrapped in his big arms. I wanted him to hold me and reassure me, with his warm and caring manner, that everything was going to be okay. Fleetingly, I imagined him helping me glue broken pieces of myself back together.

It took a great deal of determined effort to find the strength and grace to get to the table by the bar. The two men I was there to meet stood up and introduced themselves with friendly smiles.

"Nice to meet you, I'm Ruben."

"Good to meet you, I'm Rick. I know your son Marcos, and you know my ex-wife."

"Nice meeting you too," I responded, trying to be the Estela that I knew myself to be, instead of a person reeling from a cancer diagnosis.

"This is the woman who makes me smile," Jimmy said, flashing his pearly whites. That smile! I held it, a remedy for my racing heart. Ruben's wife Sandy showed up during the introductions. Her smile, too, was warm and friendly, and it helped me feel a little more at ease.

Jimmy called the waitress and ordered a Malbec. Since I'd

taken the day off, I indulged in a glass. At the first sip of the full-bodied wine, my mind drifted to Mendoza, Argentina. I hoped to visit Argentina someday to dance the tango, drink Malbec, and enjoy a steak!

Focus, I told myself.

My mind wanted to wander, rather than find its way to the topic I was avoiding. To concentrate and participate in the conversation was quite a challenge. I kept seeing numbers in my head, statistics for bilateral breast cancer.

"You like Corvettes?" Ruben asked, drawing me back into the conversation.

I answered, "Yes, I do," and he proceeded to tell me Sandy loved Corvettes. We talked about cycling, riding motorcycles, and silver and yellow Corvettes. My mind drifted away from the conversation again, multilevel thinking and compartmentalizing my thoughts into small boxes of questions in my mind.

Will I see my son graduate from high school?

Will I ever hold a grandchild in my arms?

What is Jimmy going to say?

The harder I tried to participate in the conversation, the less present I became. I knew we'd be leaving soon, and I'd get the answer to that last question. My heart was pounding, my hands were balmy, and my mouth felt like I had cotton balls stuffed in my cheeks, absorbing all of my saliva.

Jimmy noticed my discomfort and rescued me from the conversation. "Gotta go meet Estela's kids and older brother. It was great catching up!"

"Nice meeting all of you," I added.

Jimmy grabbed my hand, and we made our way out of the noisy bar and toward his truck, parked just a few feet away from the door. Nervously, I counted the steps, twenty-four in all, before Jimmy opened my door, and I jumped in. My eyes followed him as he made his way to the driver's side and opened his door. And before he could shut the door or touch the ignition switch, I opened my cotton mouth and began speaking.

"I have bilateral breast cancer. I'm having surgery on September 21st. Do you still want me to go to Asheville?"

Whew!

It all came out so fast. I made no effort to sugarcoat the truth, lie, or pretend. My anxiety was way up, feeling afraid and vulnerable, until I noticed Jimmy's green eyes open wide and teary. He grabbed my hand and held it tightly.

His voice was soft as he asked: "Do you want to stay here with your family, or do you want to come with me?"

As if the moment might pass me by, I quickly answered, "I want to go with you to Asheville."

And without skipping a beat, Jimmy began listing off the items we needed for the trip.

"You need to pack some shorts because we'll be going white water rafting, and outfits for nice dinners. You're going to love the hotel! It's magnificent," Jimmy said with a smile on his face that reached his eyes.

I gasped, feeling that sigh of relief like a rock lifted off my chest!

He didn't flinch.

He remained calm and steadfast.

You know that feeling you have? That all-of-a-sudden *knowing* that can come upon you like the first sharp rays of a sunrise in your eye? That was this moment for me.

I knew.

I knew I had just made the leap from *liking* to *loving* the man before me.

My heart was full and jumping out of my chest. He could have easily said, "I'm so sorry, but I don't think we should go on the trip. You need to be with your family," but he didn't. He could have used it as an excuse to leave me behind and go on with his life, but he didn't. Instead, he reached over the wide seat divider and held me in a deep and reassuring embrace. I melted in his arms and sobbed.

I didn't know what was going to happen next in our relationship.

It didn't matter.

I was in love, and I felt loved in return, by a man of character, who was kind and not afraid to walk with me, holding my small, bony hand in his big and strong one through whatever scary things were ahead.

For now, it was enough to know that in four days we were headed to Asheville, together.

After those tender and telling moments, we met up with my brother, Fernando, and my two oldest children, whom Jimmy had never met. What an inopportune time for him to meet my family! The five of us shared a bottle of Malbec and spoke about the uncertainty of the future. My circle of love came together to execute the action plan: a double mastectomy on September 21st and chemo to follow. Any worries I'd held about how they might get along were eased that Friday, September 1st.

As we walked out of the restaurant, Jimmy gently held my hand in his. Squeezing it tightly, he looked into my eyes, and told me and my brother, "We'll get through this together."

I reached up and hugged him, thankful for all that had passed between us that night. I placed my hands on the back of his head to help move him closer to me, and then I planted three kisses on his lips:

One kiss for promise.

One kiss for hope.

And one kiss for new love.

CHAPTER NINE

24 Words, 24 Questions, 24 Red Roses

A white rose symbolizes purity. A pink rose symbolizes grace and elegance, and a yellow rose symbolizes friendship.

A red rose is an unmistakable expression of love.

It wasn't the first time Jimmy had given me roses, but these long-stem beauties came with a deeper meaning, each velvety and fragrant petal a deep crimson. He had a tough time holding the huge bouquet, his face just peeking out from behind the green foliage and the white baby's breath.

Jimmy's forced smile, his attempt to hide his nervousness behind white teeth and deep dimples, touched my heart. He stood in the middle of the living room before slowly making his way into the kitchen, where he put down the tall bouquet. Along with the flowers, he delivered a special card from his employees, a box of chocolates from his foreman, Robert Roque, his wife Michelle, and his two children. It was such a sweet and meaningful gesture.

The last item he brought was a small white box with the symbol of a black apple. Jimmy is a thoughtful and attentive man, who, despite having so many personal and business challenges, listens to my unspoken needs and hears my heart. He knows how music lifts my spirits and gets my feet moving! Inside that small box were AirPods. He bought them for me so that in between the moments of despair and uncertainty, I could listen to music and sing along to my favorite songs from Adele, Sam Smith, Sara Bareilles, and Luis Miguel. Their soothing voices could block all the noise in my head and calm my fears about facing the next steps.

Each of the 24 roses represented special words in my heart as I prepared for surgery the following morning. Love, hope, fear, anxiety, faith, strength, courage, grit, uncertainty, promise, kindness, gratitude, trust, vanity, pride, dedication, commitment, integrity, drive, growth, family, happiness, relief, and determination.

My brain echoed with the questions I was facing:

Will the surgeon be able to remove ALL the cancer?

Will the surgery be more extensive?

Is there a chance I could die on the operating table?

Will Dr. Landeros find something unexpected when he gets a clear view of my breasts?

What will the pathology show?

Will there be cancer in the lymph nodes?

Will the pain be unbearable?

What will I look like after?

Will I still have a good range of motion?

Will I need physical therapy?

Will Jimmy still like me with fake breasts?

What about my children? Will they be embarrassed that everyone knows their mother has implants?

How will I feel when I look in the mirror?

Is there a chance my scars will get infected?

When can I go back to work?

Will others define me by my cancer diagnosis?

How will people look at me?

Will my clothes still fit?

How will I face the challenges ahead?

What are the statistics after a double mastectomy?

What if the implants end up being too big?

I knew the AirPods would come in handy to still the noise in my mind, but it was the presence of Jimmy, my son Marcos, Ana, my longtime housekeeper, and the prayers and positive vibes around me that brought me peace that evening.

The sweet reassurance came when Jimmy leaned over and kissed me with trembling lips. We would fight this together. Juntos.

CHAPTER TEN

Dancing in the Rain

It was still dark at 5:00 a.m. when Jimmy picked me up to head to the airport. We were both feeling giddy as we boarded the flight to Atlanta and then on to Asheville. We were in the 14th row of the airplane; it was a tight squeeze for Jimmy since he's so tall! His knees hit the seat in front of us. I lifted the armrest between us. He held my hand, and I rested my head on his shoulder. We were both looking forward to this time away together, without the disruptions of work and family. It was a first for us. How would we get along for 96 hours straight?

We were both emotionally exhausted, so getting away and leaving behind all the tragic news was welcome. As the plane lifted off the runway and above the clouds, our cares lifted too. We both kept dozing off, thanks to our very early start, but our hands remained intertwined.

After we had to change planes several times and enjoyed a few quick naps, we eventually made it into Asheville. A driver at the airport, holding a piece of paper with our names, whisked us away to the hotel. We enjoyed a twenty-minute tour of the city before making our way to the hotel. It was magnificent, just as Jimmy had promised.

The Omni Grove Hotel was built in 1913 and sits atop Sunset Mountain within the Blue Ridge Mountains. It's listed on the National Register of Historic Places. The facade is assembled with rocks and crowned with a red roof. The hotel is surrounded by a golf course and a manicured lawn. Many famous people have stayed there, including ten US presidents and author F. Scott Fitzgerald. It took my breath away!

Before heading to our room, we explored the grounds, checking out the different restaurants and gift shops. Flames danced in a massive fireplace with a wide hearth in the lobby. I stopped to listen to the crackling of the firewood, enchanted with it all, feeling so grateful to be able to have this time with Jimmy. And then, there he was again, taking my hand and leading me to our room, where the magic of the moment lived on. A spectacular view of the golf course and the Blue Ridge Mountains awaited us in the room. Light fog billowed in the North Carolina air. We opened the window to let in the light breeze and to smell the fresh air. Breathing it in felt like peace.

I had packed several nice outfits, and I decided on a black dress and five-inch heels for our special dinner in the ballroom that evening. I'm five foot one, and I need the extra height to look into Jimmy's eyes.

"Can you please help me with my necklace?" I asked, putting the finishing touches on my look.

Jimmy got behind me and carefully placed the silver statement necklace on my neck. I felt my body tingle, responding to the light brush of his lips on the nape. I turned around and gave him our signature three kisses before dabbing on some lipstick. (Side note: Always, ALWAYS make time for those kisses!) I helped him finish buttoning his crisply pressed lavender-colored shirt. He looked very handsome with his navy slacks, dress shoes, and belt with a silver buckle. With his big smile and deep dimples, he looked like a dream come to life. I sighed in contentment, admiring him standing in front of me.

We made our way downstairs to the patio for martinis before joining the group for the buffet dinner. I wasn't very hungry, but we enjoyed the food and especially the desserts! We took in the tunes played by the folk band for a bit; then we decided to explore the grounds at dusk.

It was a damp night in Asheville, and the steps at the Omni were wet and slippery, especially in stilettos! I held tight to Jimmy's arm as it began to sprinkle. As we made our way down the stairs to check out the spa at the bottom of the hotel, the live music from the ballroom blared, echoing down to our ears.

Feeling adventurous, and in love, I asked Jimmy, "Mr. Dick, can I have this dance?"

His answer to that invitation needed no words. He took my right hand in his and grabbed my waist, pulling me into his arms. I put my head on his chest, and we danced right there in the rain, taking the time to be fully present together in that magical moment.

There's a saying: "The person who dances with you in the rain will be with you in the storm." The trip to Asheville marked a defining moment in our relationship and cancer journey. In my heart, I felt the storm ahead, but as we danced under the night sky, awash in light raindrops, I knew everything was going to be okay. We were making magic together, and it was just the first night!

Our adventures for the next day included white water rafting. That morning, as I excitedly zipped up my wetsuit, and Jimmy tied his tennis shoes, my phone rang. Dr. Mark Landeros's name flashed on the screen. My heart began to pound in my chest as I looked at Jimmy and answered it, putting the phone on speaker.

"This is Dr. Landeros. I called to let you know I've received the complete pathology report. The third test shows you have HER2 positive breast cancer. We have to postpone the double mastectomy. You need to start chemotherapy right away."

His words, heavy words, intruded.

"You will get the first of 6 rounds on September 14th, with an additional 12 rounds of Herceptin, an immunotherapy drug. It's an aggressive cancer, and we have to treat it aggressively," he concluded.

I listened quietly, the weight of those words rooting me to the chair and echoing through my mind.

HER2 positive. Postpone. Chemotherapy. Herceptin.

Aggressive.

Aggressive.

AGGRESSIVE.

In shock, I said, "Dr. Landeros, that's some devastating news. I'm out of town through the 8th."

He answered, "Then the 14th is perfect to start the treatment. I'll contact Dr. Valilis to set up your treatment protocol. We'll get you through this. I'm sorry."

I'm sorry.

"We'll get through this; thank you, Doctor," I replied.

Jimmy stood next to me, tears standing in his eyes. He didn't speak. I didn't either; we felt that time stood still. The news was grim.

Oh, my God! What now?

Despite my own emerging tears, I held it together. I held it together because we were out of town together. I held it together because I had promised myself that I would enjoy every moment of our time together. I felt terrified, but I held it together, because I was determined not to let the cancer make me wallow in fear or pity—especially at a time when I just wanted to be enjoying myself and my love.

Jimmy gave me his hand and pulled me up off the chair. He wiped my tears, gave me a quick slap on the butt, and told me to get ready. I ran to the bathroom to lather on some sunblock, apply some waterproof mascara, and kept getting ready for our big adventure.

It was a beautiful day in North Carolina, perfect for white water rafting. The cloudless sky was open, and fresh breezes teased our skin. I was, in truth, a little nervous about our outing. I'm not a strong swimmer, and I was deathly afraid of the water, but I felt safe with Jimmy. The river was calm and smooth, the water warm. We were surrounded by beautiful views and deep blue water. Our boat went through several bends and currents, and the ride was exhilarating!

We enjoyed four glorious days in Asheville getting to know each other on a deeper, more spiritual level. We decided not to discuss my diagnosis or prognosis. It simply wasn't the time.

Reality hit hard when we arrived back home. The team assembled, ready or not, to hit the ground running, knowing the cancer was aggressive. I knew I wasn't alone in the fight, but the journey ahead was still daunting.

I worked to strengthen my relationships with the most important people in my life. I began strengthening my relationship with God. He was tugging at my ear to remind me who was in charge.

I surrendered.

And I made Him a promise:

"I will do the best I can. I will follow doctor's orders and live life to the fullest, but you're in charge of the rest. *Lord, make me an instrument of your peace.* Show me what else I, and my circle of love, need to do to get through the process. My heart is open to receive. My soul, ripe to fill."

My head?

Well, I had to work on that!

CHAPTER ELEVEN

Perfect Sunday

Our hearts were ringing
In the key that our souls were singing
As we danced in the night
Remember how the stars stole the night away
Hey hey hey
Ba de ya, say do you remember?
Ba de ya, dancing in September
Ba de ya, never was a cloudy day

From: "September" by Earth, Wind & Fire

September is one of my most favorite months. The afternoons are cooler, and the evenings produce stunning sunsets in the southwest. September is also my son Andres' birthday month.

He was born on September 9th, but 14 is a milestone, so we celebrated his 14th birthday every time we went out to eat that year!

One of our favorite celebrations happened at Sandra's house. She'd invited Andres, Marcos, and me to swim and to throw some burgers on the grill. Sandra has a party friendly backyard with an outdoor kitchen and a saltwater pool and jacuzzi. Our friend Toni, and her eight-year-old son Gregory, also came over to help blow out some candles.

We were also using the opportunity for Team Estela to strategize on the pool deck with some tequila and music. The sky was a wide, clear blue, and it matched the water in the pool. The colors around me seemed more vibrant and alive. The boys jumped in, but instead of splashing in the water, they floated on foam tubes. Unlike most days, they were eerily quiet. Andres kept looking at me, smiling.

But Marcos!

Marcos didn't smile. His eyes didn't sparkle, and his normally open face was somber.

Marcos understood what lay ahead for me—and for us as a family. He saw the consequences of breast cancer in his workplace. He was working as a physical therapy tech in one of Sandra's clinics. Some of the women he helped to gain mobility had battled breast cancer. They had shared their stories with him, of the challenges of not being able to move after a mastectomy. He showed them stretching exercises so they could regain strength and become more agile and mobile. As I observed him, glancing at everything around him with his sad eyes and somber expression, I felt a pang of guilt. My boys were hurting, and I wished I could take away their pain and suffering.

Marcos had just completed four years of college in Kirksville, Missouri and had come home. He'd decided to take a year off to work, and then apply to a physical therapy program later. I was *not* happy that he was taking a year off before enrolling in graduate school. I thought taking a break would distract him from reaching his end goal. That year off actually turned into only a few months off when he was accepted into the University of Texas at El Paso Doctor of Physical Therapy Program. He would be staying in El Paso and starting classes immediately.

As usual, God knew better than I. He knew I needed Marcos at home. God-Incidence? Absolutely! As the boys floated in the saltwater pool that Sunday afternoon, I marveled how God and cancer were transforming their lives, changing them—and us—forever.

There at Sandra's, the magic was strong, creating special moments and memories under the September sun. We basked in the sunlight in tankinis and bikinis.

It took cancer to make me realize I looked pretty good in a bathing suit. Working out at the gym for many years had toned my arms and legs. But I'd never felt my waistline was small enough, my butt round enough, or my breasts perky enough.

I never thought I was enough.

Facing a possible death sentence made me realize that I am enough. Those flaws and idiosyncrasies I'd agonized over for years were not more important than me loving myself. I realized I should not be ashamed of showing my waistline, which had expanded after giving birth to three children. It showed that I was woman enough to create life! My breasts had shrunk as cancer began attacking them, but those same breasts had successfully nursed three babies, because I *am* enough.

I knew that, in the battle ahead, I wasn't going to have time to worry about how my body looked. I would have to depend on it to be strong and ready for the chemotherapy that was just a few days away.

But that day! That day was for joy and celebration.

There were hotdogs, hamburgers, potato chips, and an assortment of munchies. And there was a lot to drink!

As the tequila started flowing, so did the tears and cheers. As we raised our shot glasses with tequila Patrón, we toasted to life! We yelled, "Salud!" in unison. We shared stories and laughed so hard our bellies and cheeks ached. We yelled, "Fuck cancer!" and raised our glasses to fight together. "Salud!"

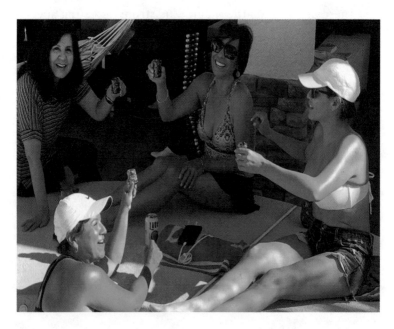

We posed for pictures on the deck. Marcos snapped some candid shots that captured love, laughter, family, and friendship. It was a glorious evening, filled with unforgettable and poignant moments. Cancer made us pivot; made me search for, and find, all the magic in my life. There was so much magic around me . . . that we helped create.

Our conversations and laughter were suddenly drowned by the sound of trumpets, violins, guitars, and strong, beautiful voices. Mariachi band members began parading in from the side gate and into the backyard! Sandra had hired them just for us.

What a treat! Music always makes me feel better. It's the universal language of love, and that day, it also turned into a language of hope. We sang a few songs, casting our hopes into the air itself.

In less than 24 hours, on September 11th, I would officially begin my cancer journey, by having a port-a-cath (a device that puts a tube in the vena cava to deliver chemotherapy directly into the heart) placed while under general anesthesia. It was about to get real, the path ahead, uncertain. Chemotherapy and surgery were the only options for me, and neither had any guarantee of success.

But I wasn't going to borrow worry, yet.

The sun was setting in the autumn sky as the mariachis picked up their instruments and left. We all got in the pool. I grabbed a floaty and allowed my body to relax and enjoy the warm water.

The calm before the storm.

The perfect Sunday!

CHAPTER TWELVE

Bright Yellow Socks

Where were you on September 11, 2001?

Everyone I know remembers exactly where they were, and what they were doing as the world watched the Twin Towers go down. We recall in painfully exquisite detail, the roller coaster of emotions we all experienced, as we realized nearly three thousand Americans had been killed in the coordinated attacks of that day.

I normally didn't watch TV in the early morning because I was too busy trying to get the kids ready for school. But that morning, for some reason, I turned on the TV in our bedroom. And when the images came up, I couldn't move. I remember feeling helpless and unsafe, wondering if our community was next. It would be a natural place to carry out an attack: Fort Bliss, Biggs Field, White Sands, and Holloman Air Force Base are all in close proximity. I stood frozen, watching the anchors and reporters attempting to make sense of it all. They searched for words to explain to viewers what they were seeing unfold, with no words adequate for the job.

Everything changed that day.

Fast forward sixteen years.

At right around the same time, 6:45 a.m. El Paso time, Marcos and I headed to the Hospitals of Providence Memorial campus for the outpatient procedure to insert the port-a-cath to deliver chemo into my body.

Marcos hit the ground running toward his doctoral program at UTEP, and he had a test he couldn't miss that morning. After we registered, and I settled in behind the curtains in a small corner of pre-op, I insisted he leave.

"I'll be okay, Papi. Good luck on your test and I'll see you in the afternoon after Toni takes me home," I said in a soft voice so no one could hear behind curtains two and three.

Marcos smiled and said: "I'll see you at the house. Love you."

Behind curtain number one, I found myself alone with my thoughts, a hum of indistinguishable conversations around me. I tuned them out, praying and gathering my courage, sporting a lovely thin blue cap and gray gown with small designs and clips on the shoulders that opened to the backside.

My nurse popped her head behind curtain number one, and said cheerily, "Good morning, Ms. Casas! I have some special socks to keep your feet warm." The warmth in her smile lit her up as she continued, "They're yellow—the color of sunshine!"

The smiles were infectious, and the socks were everything she promised: warm, fuzzy, and slip free!

Turning her attention from the socks, and holding a notebook and pen, she started on a litany of questions.

"Are you allergic to any medications? Are you pregnant? Do you have a living will?" she asked.

"No, no, yes," I answered, listening to the *scratch, scratch, scratch* of her pen as she wrote down my answers.

A defining and sobering moment came when the nurse asked me what side the port-a-cath was going in.

"We can put it on the side that doesn't have the tumor," she told me confidently.

But her expression changed when I answered, "I have tumors in both breasts."

It didn't matter where the port would be located.

This is a little technical, but I will explain in layman's terms. The port-a-cath is a device that's implanted below the skin in the chest area just below the collarbone. It is attached to a long catheter that is threaded into the large vein above the right side of the heart, called the superior vena cava. The device was going to save me several needle pricks during chemo. I would only get one prick, and the chemo would be delivered directly into the heart to help the drugs circulate more quickly and effectively.

The pre-op area smelled like all hospitals do, clean and disinfected, with the stale air of sterility. It was abuzz with patients and their families. Although Marcos had left, I wasn't alone for long, as several people came in to say hello. Some wore scrubs, and others wore suits.

The Hospitals of Providence CEO, Sally Hurt-Deitch, is a good friend. She was out of town, but she sent three top administrators to welcome me and to reassure me I was in good hands. I picked up on the expressions on their faces; their forced smiles communicated their concern and compassion. They were glad I chose their hospital, but they weren't happy to see me under those circumstances. They were used to seeing me in a suit and high heels, delivering speeches or emceeing functions. They were used to seeing me in full makeup and delivering the nightly news. Instead, that morning, they found me looking vulnerable and scared.

Dr. Landeros showed up in gray scrubs and a surgical cap.

"Good morning, Estela; how are you feeling?" he asked.

With a raspy voice I had lost while singing and laughing the night before, I answered, "I'm here, doctor; let's get the party started."

He reassured me the procedure under general anesthesia would be quick, but he still warned that I would feel a little sore in the morning. I felt myself dozing off, and the next thing I knew, I was in recovery with a bandage on the left side of my chest, a round object under my skin, my badge of honor, and the warm yellow socks on my feet.

The journey began on September 11th. My personal 9/11. My life, and the lives of my loved ones, would be forever changed.

CHAPTER THIRTEEN

See This Through Together

"It's the 7th of the month, time to Keep Abreast of your health and do a monthly self-exam. Get in front of a mirror and check for changes and use your middle and index fingers to check for lumps. If you noticed any changes, make an appointment to see your doctor. Remember, early detection saves lives."

For many years at KVIA I delivered that message. Many years before that, as the main anchor at KDBC-TV, I spearheaded the Texas Breast Cancer Screening Project. I'd been an advocate of breast cancer awareness for longer than some of my colleagues had been alive!

My circle of love knew about my diagnosis and the execution of my care plan. Now I had the tough challenge of sharing that information with those colleagues and with the community of El Paso. The public journey was about to get underway and I was feeling a little uneasy. How would people react? Was I ready for putting this public face on my very personal journey?

Despite struggling with these questions, I headed out the door to work, feeling (for the moment) confident in my decision to fight this battle publicly. When I walked into my office, I found two dozen red roses on my desk, taking up most of the available space. I opened the card that was secured in a plastic holder. It said:

"Always remember 95%. We will see this through together. JD."

What a way to start the day! Those words from my BMAC, Jimmy, gave me the strength and courage to find the appropriate words to share with my coworkers and viewers.

Everyone in the newsroom began taking their seats at the conference table for our editorial meeting. I walked in and sat in my designated seat at the edge of the big brown table. I looked out the glass windows with Jimmy's encouraging words in my mind. Then I took a deep breath, looked over at KVIA-TV News Director Brenda De Anda Swann for approval, and began to speak.

"Tomorrow I will have my first of six chemotherapy treatments. I have bilateral breast cancer and will later have a double mastectomy."

Saying those life-changing words out loud was humbling! I started to tremble. I skimmed the room, noticing how everyone had started squirming. They didn't know how to react to the news. Some stared at me, others looked down. Most teared up to varying degrees.

I continued, "I apologize for adding any extra work to your

schedule because I will be going in every 21 days for treatment and will be missing work. I am ready to fight with your help. I will make an announcement on the air today."

Have you ever tried smiling with tears in your eyes? It's hard when they're not happy tears, but I did it. The room remained silent as I pushed back my chair from the table, got up, and walked back into my office. My steps were strong and deliberate. In a very real way, I felt I was marking the steps I would take in this journey, letting everyone around me know I was able for this journey, and it was starting right now. The two-week old secret was out. My shoulders felt lighter as I sat back down in my office, reading Jimmy's note one more time.

I now had the task of taking my thoughts and feelings, and putting all of it on paper to tell my story. I felt the weight of tremendous responsibility to my viewers. How would I tell them about my fight with breast cancer?

I answered my own question with honesty and clarity.

CHAPTER FOURTEEN

Mi Verdad

It didn't take long for the word to spread to the other side of the building. It seemed like only moments before coworkers from sales, administration, and production began parading into my office to offer their support and comfort. The newsroom, usually abuzz with noise, remained silent as producers and reporters stayed at their desks and on their computers. While working to crank out the news of the day, they were processing the information themselves before sharing it with their own family and friends.

News deadlines have to be met no matter what's going on in our world. Once the camera light flashes green, it's showtime! Only an hour into the evening shift, I was already emotionally drained. It had been tough sharing my devastating news in the editorial meeting. It got tougher as I kept having to repeat the story to everyone who came to my office or called my desk.

I finally chose to stop answering both my personal and work phones. I had hourly deadlines to meet for writing, reading over, and editing scripts for the early newscasts. I couldn't let the chaos in either my environment, or my brain, keep me from writing the script I would be sharing during the 10 p.m. newscast.

At first, I just put my hands on the keyboard and let my brain tell my fingers the words and sentences to form across the keypad. I only had two minutes allotted to tell this story. I rewrote it several times. As tough as the writing process was, the biggest challenge was still ahead. My mind raced with questions.

Can I deliver this news to my viewers with grace? Can I keep it together enough to tell this story with dignity?

The mascara I'd been wearing inevitably wound up in a tissue. I reapplied it, swept more rouge on my cheeks, and dabbed on a glossy lipstick. I adjusted my mind *and* my flowered zip-up blazer and delivered the 5 and 6 p.m. newscasts, as if nothing were wrong. As though my life wasn't shifting right before everyone's eyes. I got through it all. We all got through the day.

At 9:45 p.m., after looking over all the scripts I was assigned to read, I headed to the restroom to gather my thoughts. I clutched the pages like a rosary, praying for strength. My heart beat so hard and fast, I thought people must be able to hear it! My palms were sweating, and I felt breathless.

Please, God, help me get through this announcement without breaking down, I prayed in silence.

I walked into the studio with firm, steady steps. My coanchor, Rick Cabrera, was already on set. He looked up from the laptop he was typing on and said, "You're ready. I'm here for you."

I smiled, adjusted my chair, clipped on the lavalier micro-phone, and took a deep breath that turned into a sigh of relief. All of a sudden, I felt at peace, knowing I was no longer hiding a secret.

We read the top news stories of the day, and then Rick tossed it to me, saying, "You have some personal news you'd like to share."

I turned to my designated camera and began speaking and sharing my truth:

"BLESSINGS COME IN DIFFERENT FORMS.
MINE CAME LAST MONTH AFTER I GOT A TETANUS SHOT.
THAT BUMP THAT FORMED IN MY RIGHT ARM FORCED ME TO THE DOCTOR'S OFFICE AND A DEV-ASTATING DIAGNOSIS.
AFTER REPORTING ON BREAST CANCER FOR MORE THAN THREE DECADES, I JOIN MILLIONS OF WOMEN AND MEN FIGHTING AGAINST THIS POTEN-TIALLY DEADLY DISEASE.
YOU'VE NOTICED THAT I'VE LOST WEIGHT, I HADN'T FELT THIS GOOD IN SUCH A LONG TIME.
BUT LOOKS ARE DECEIVING.
I HAVE BILATERAL BREAST CANCER.
TOMORROW, I BEGIN MY CANCER JOURNEY.
I WILL BE ADMINISTERED THE FIRST ROUND OF CHEMOTHERAPY.
YOU WILL SEE SOME CHANGES IN MY APPEARANCE, BUT MY PASSION FOR MY JOB WILL NOT CHANGE.

GETTING THAT TETANUS SHOT WAS A BLESSING IN DISGUISE.

I WILL BE TAKING SOME TIME OFF A FEW DAYS A MONTH TO FIGHT THE GOOD FIGHT LIKE SO MANY OTHER WOMEN IN OUR COMMUNITY!

I HAVE A STRONG AND COMPASSIONATE TEAM OF FAMILY, FRIENDS, DOCTORS, BOSSES, AND COWORKERS WHO WILL BE WITH ME ON THIS CANCER JOURNEY.

BUT MORE IMPORTANTLY I HAVE TURNED IT OVER TO GOD.

I WOULD GREATLY APPRECIATE YOUR PRAYERS."*

*Actual script

In between all these words, short breaths, and pauses, my eyes swelled with tears. My voice began to tremble, but I pulled through.

What a relief it was to stop carrying the weight of my story, my secret struggle. I had given myself permission to fight. My public battle with bilateral breast cancer began that very moment. I unclipped my microphone, gave Rick a hug, walked off the set, and headed to the bathroom to gather my things.

With tears in my eyes, I collected the lipstick, loose powder, brushes, and hairspray, and stuffed it all in the cosmetic bag. I slipped out of the station quietly, even before the newscast was over, walked to my car, and drove home.

I'd received so much love and support from everyone by that

point, that it was hard to be struck with a sobering truth:

Although we are surrounded by well-wishes, love, and caring, we ultimately fight alone . . . with our thoughts, alone with our heart, and alone with our God.

CHAPTER FIFTEEN

Red Convertible

Buzzz . . . buzzzz . . .

The vibration of my phone announced that it was 6:00 a.m.

It was also my reminder that it was the first day of chemotherapy.

Before I flung over the sheet on the bed, I opened my Facebook messenger to read the prayer of the day from St. Luke's Catholic Church. That day's prayer was longer because it included my intentions.

I jumped out of bed and into the shower. I let the warm water run over my body, and I followed its progress to my toes as my brain shifted into overdrive.

What will I feel when the chemo drugs start running through my veins?

How will my body react to the poison?

Will my body be able to carry me through the treatment?

I gave myself a pep talk, reminding myself that through the years, I had been making good food choices, staying active with spinning classes, doing Zumba, and lifting weights. My heart was strong and healthy from the cardio workouts. I was in good shape physically and in a good place emotionally. My heart and soul felt ready.

I got out of the shower, towel-dried, and slipped on a sports bra, black yoga pants, pink socks with bright letters that read "Fight like a Girl," tennis shoes, and a pink shirt Sandra had bought for me to wear. My "chemo day" bag was stocked with water, snacks, an iPad, a blanket, and lipstick. I'm a firm believer in never leaving the house without lipstick!

Sandra arrived in her red convertible Mercedes Benz and a heart full of hope and caring.

"Buenos días," she said with a smile.

"Buenos días," I responded. "Let's do this!"

I was riding to my first treatment in style. I climbed in, Sandra revved the engine, and we sped away from the neighborhood. We didn't put the top down. We should have!

We laughed during the twenty-minute drive to downtown, making small talk. As we made our way down Mesa Street, Sandra slowed down and turned into a private parking lot across from St. Patrick Cathedral.

"Let's go in so you can say a prayer and take communion," Sandra said, knowing I needed a spiritual boost to kick off this journey into the unknown.

Parishioners were walking out and hugging Father Trini, who

was in a green robe in the back of the cathedral. I, too, gave him a hug and told him why I was there. He already knew, and he led me to the front of the church. As I walked up the side aisle, I felt the icons follow me to the sacristy. They knew I was there to ask for special intentions. God knew I was there to ask for his blessing.

Father Trini said a prayer and offered the Eucharist. I had stopped going to church two years before, when my husband and I separated. I hadn't gone to confession or communion during that time, either. I'd only been divorced for three months, and I didn't feel worthy to partake. Strictly speaking, I wasn't at that moment, but that day, I felt assured God would make an exception. I knelt in one of the pews and opened my heart, asking for His forgiveness, grace, and blessing; then I extended my cupped hands and received the host. I prayed as it melted inside my mouth. I felt God's peace knowing He would be holding my hand during this journey.

"Thank you, Father Trini," Sandra and I said in unison.

Filled with faith, encouragement, and hope, we arrived at Texas Oncology on Grandview. I had been to the building before, but this time was different. I was throwing the first punch in my fight against cancer, stepping into the space where we all were fighting to stay alive with IVs connected to our bodies.

"Good morning, Ms. Casas, please stop by the lab before you head to the second floor. The nurses are waiting for you," said the receptionist.

I had some blood drawn, and then we headed to the elevator.

Let me tell you about these nurses! I noticed many of them smiling a lot. I admired them for being able to do that, because although I'm told being an oncology nurse is rewarding, it also can take a hard toll. They establish a friendship with a patient they see every three weeks, or even every day, only to learn later that they lost their battle. I imagined them as guardian angels, watching over people in need of care.

"Good morning," my nurse greeted us, leading us to another room.

He took my weight, blood pressure, oxygen, and pulse. My pressure was a little high for my liking, but within the normal range.

"Your vitals are good. You can go to the other room and settle down on one of our comfy recliners," he said with a reassuring smile. "I'm so sorry you're going through this, but we'll get through this together."

I smiled back, and said, "We will, so let's do this!"

I took firm steps down the hall to the infusion center. My eyes skimmed the room, and I noticed an empty recliner in the far-left corner. I claimed it for myself. It was near a window, so I could enjoy the outside view, and still watch television if I wanted to. Sandra and I pulled everything out of the chemo bag, arranging the items it contained all around the area to make it more inviting.

The room was a little chilly, so I draped a light blanket over my legs. As I busied myself with that, another nurse rolled over the chemo-cart containing several IV bags. She explained that I was going to be administered double doses of carboplatin and docetaxel, which are chemotherapy drugs for HER2 positive breast cancer, and two immunotherapy targeted drugs: Herceptin and Perjeta. I had already taken two days of steroids pills to avoid an allergic reaction. I was given anti-nausea and anti-anxiety medications and two painkillers.

"Ms. Casas, this first session will last about nine hours because we need to make sure you'll be okay with all the new medications in your system," said the nurse.

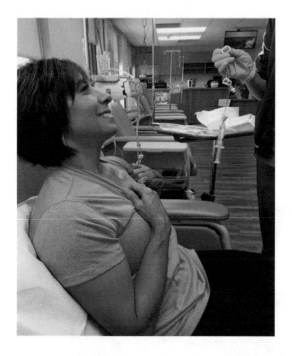

The meds knocked me out for quite a bit of those nine hours. I drifted in and out of sleep. All those drugs will do that! Patients started coming in, staking out their spots to receive treatment. I traded smiles and greetings with them when I wasn't asleep. Sandra brought lunch and made sure I was drinking water to stay hydrated. I wasn't very hungry, but I forced myself to eat. For the rest of that nine hours, I got on social media, read a book, watched TV, and planned for the future, even though I wondered if I would even have one. It looked so uncertain.

Sandra was my touchstone that day. She kept me entertained as we laughed, checked emails and voice messages, and monitored Facebook, Instagram, Twitter, and LinkedIn. I felt blessed listening to the voice messages viewers left and reading hundreds of messages on social media. I was surrounded by love and prayers. How could I not be positive and hopeful? That army of prayer warriors, including people I didn't even know! (¡Pequeños milagros!), was going to get me through the toughest fight of my life.

I need to say, also, that I believe in medication and using all the medical tools and advances available to me. But I still had to turn myself over to God. That's really all I could do.

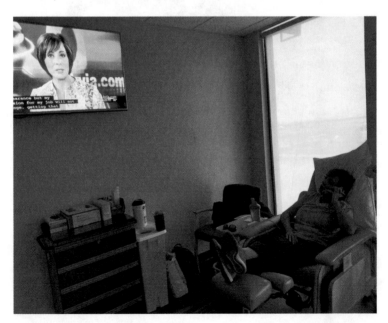

Soon afterward, it was time to go home in the red convertible again. A bright half-moon shined brightly on us in the early evening sky, and the soft breeze blew through our hair. I imagined how the poison of chemo was blowing through my veins, hopefully doing the work of helping to rid my body of cancer. And I thought about those prayers I had asked for, and how I'd received that and so much more.

Viewers sent in flowers, blankets, T-shirts, books, blessed rosaries from Fatima, Portugal, holy water from Mexico, and holy soil from Chimayo, New Mexico, which means sanctuary. Hundreds of thousands of believers make pilgrimages to the small town near Taos, New Mexico to scoop up the red healing soil. Chimayo is located in the foothills of the Sangre de Cristo Mountains and is a National Historic Landmark. The sanctuary is one of the most important Catholic pilgrimage centers in the United States.

All week I received thousands of emails, comments, and phone calls from people in the Borderland, and from people with connections to El Paso, Las Cruces, and Ciudad Juarez. My community had lifted me and my family in prayer and love, and my heart was full and grateful.

CHAPTER SIXTEEN

Faith in Motion

While hooked up to the IV in the infusion center, I got a call from KVIA general manager, Kevin Lovell. Kevin told me he had received a call from Nancy Keane of Albertsons, saying she wanted to donate $50,000 in my name to cancer patients! I knew of Nancy but had not met her but she knew about my love for my community.

Remember those small miracles I mentioned before? Here was where they became the big one!

Nancy had provided the seed money. My dear Sandra offered a vision for what it could become, and mean, for the community. Sandra and I had talked about it during the long hours during chemo and in between my naps. Jimmy offered a vehicle to get it started. He made some phone calls and arranged a high-powered meeting in his boardroom with the President and CEO of the El

Paso Community Foundation, Eric Pearson. My coworkers at KVIA rallied behind the project and it quickly came together as the "Stand with Estela" fund under the El Paso Community Foundation.

I believe with all my heart that there are always angels around us to help guide us through the challenges we face in life. We just have to have an open heart and mind to acknowledge and honor their presence. Nancy's offer made her one of those angels who helped get me and my family through the cancer process.

Before I knew it, news releases were issued to print and broadcast media to announce the creation of the Stand with Estela fund.

My friend Toni drove me to the Foundation room of the El Paso Community Foundation. It was standing room only when she and I walked in, and I was in complete and utter shock at the sight! Emotions came at me fast as I took in the cameras, microphones, and mountains of wires belonging to TV, radio, and print reporters. The room was filled with faces both familiar and not, but they all flashed friendly smiles and gave warm handshakes, hugs, and air kisses.

There was electricity in the air! That may sound like an exaggeration, but it's exactly how it played out. It's rare, *unheard of*, to fill a room of media from television, radio, and newspaper to cover a project or announcement from a competing station. Their presence there signaled something much bigger than competing for viewers. And even though it was the Stand with Estela fund, I just happened to be the conduit.

I tried to acknowledge everyone in the room, all my friends and former coworkers. I smiled and thanked them, but their faces became blurry the closer I got to the front of the room, determined to make this moment count.

I skimmed the room and found my son, Marcos. He was shaking hands and thanking people for supporting our family, but his hazel-colored eyes were zeroed in on me. I smiled, waved, and mouthed, "*I love you,*" as I wondered what he was thinking. I hoped that in the middle of all the tragedy, he could feel proud of his mama, understanding why I had to fight this battle in public. He'd taken the afternoon off from his work as a PT tech to celebrate with me and be my strength, hands in the pockets of his black scrubs.

My girlfriends, Sandra, Nicole, Toni, Griselda, and Margie, were there too. I could feel their energy, love, and sisterhood. Sandra, Nicole, and Toni came into my life at different times for different reasons. Griselda and Margie have been lifelong friends. All of them are angels who have guided me and my family during some difficult times in our lives. Some cancer sisters were there too. I could sense the quiet strength of their presence.

Looking out further, I found my tall and handsome Jimmy. He was sporting a blue and white checkered shirt and navy pants. He stood proudly and flashed a smile that highlighted his deep dimples. My breath caught, as I noticed he was wearing the pink bracelet stamped with Stand with Estela on his left wrist. He, as much as anyone there, was a big reason why the room was full. Everyone else in the room disappeared as we locked eyes, mine saying, "Thank you," and his responding, "I'm here for you."

KVIA News Director Brenda de Anda-Swann and station engineers were busy setting up cameras and microphones and taking in the excitement of the unprecedented event.

My boss, KVIA General Manager Kevin Lovell, whom I've known for more than twenty years, wore a coat and tie. Kevin doesn't always wear a tie, but that day was special. He was holding a check from News Press and Gazette, which owns KVIA. Sitting next to him were Nancy Keane, from Albertsons, and Sally Hurt-Deitch from the Hospitals of Providence. They, too, were holding big checks with lots of zeroes!

Beloved El Paso icon Rosa Guerrero also sat in the first row, sending love and blessings. Rosa holds a special place in my heart. She's a mother figure who transmits love when she holds your hands in hers. I know what she means to me, and what I mean to her, and that gift is immeasurable.

KVIA's general sales manager, Kalvin Pike, observed in amazement. He was new to the station, and to El Paso. Such an effort and gathering was unprecedented.

Unprecedented, but also maybe unsurprising in the Sun City, where family is more than just a word or concept, and includes bonds forged with or without blood relation. Former coworkers, now competitors, news anchors, and reporters from other stations, from print, from radio, from El Paso, and from across the border, weren't just there to cover a story. They were there supporting a friend and colleague.

Robert Holguin from KFOX14 was there with that twinkle in his eye. Don Guevara from KTSM had sent me a bouquet of flowers when I first made my announcement, and he stood there that day in support. Former coworker Shelton Dotson, who was now at CBS, brought me a dozen pink roses, beautiful and fragrant! He placed the roses in my arms, hugged me, and said, "I love you," with tears in his eyes.

We came, united in purpose, to inform our viewers, listeners, and readers that we had created a fund to help women with fewer resources fight cancer. To announce that breast cancer in our community had a new face. It had a new and bilingual voice. The room was abuzz with activity and conversation. It was magical. My eyes glazed over in awe and tears.

I wore a black jersey blouse with bell sleeves and a cutout in the chest area. I pinned a sparkly rhinestone pink ribbon above my left breast. The black and white skirt was tight-fitting and just above my knees. My shoes were black with leather laces wrapped around the ankles. I wore a black leather belt, white beaded earrings, and a smile.

I remember exactly what I wore, and I chose that outfit because I wanted to let people know that despite the cancer growing inside my chest, I still felt beautiful. Women need to be reminded that they have inner beauty, and they need to allow it to radiate, no matter what's going on in their lives.

Cancer is real, very real, but the mind is a powerful tool you need in your arsenal. Fighting cancer is a mind game. I don't like to play games, but I wasn't about to lose the biggest and most challenging one of my life. I was under the lights and on stage learning how to play and win against this terrifying disease. I had no choice but to present myself the only way I knew how—in control and confident.

After a beautiful introduction from Erik Pearson, the executive director of the El Paso Community Foundation, I got behind the podium. Cameras, recording devices, and microphones started rolling and recording. I stood in front of the beautiful green backdrop and opened my mouth to speak, but it sounded soft and shaky to my ears.

I felt overwhelmed, but I found my voice again in embracing my vulnerability and speaking my truth. I shared intimate details about battling breast cancer and thanked those who prayed for me. I asked my community to share that love they showed me with others who are less fortunate. I asked them to share their time, their talent, and their treasure with women who, unlike me, lacked the support and resources to fight this ruthless disease.

Community in motion.

Faith in motion.

Love in motion.

Small miracles, indeed.

CHAPTER SEVENTEEN

Have a Pink Day!

Life was moving quickly; with so much activity at home and at work, I didn't have time to ponder my illness. But two weeks after my first chemo treatment, four days after announcing the Stand with Estela fund and with my second chemotherapy treatment looming, I was feeling discombobulated.

My body was beginning to feel the effects of the poison seeping into every pore in my body, running through my veins and organs, chomping away at the cancer cells dividing in my breasts. I had a metallic taste in my mouth all the time. I was nauseated a lot; my stomach churned no matter what I did—or didn't—eat.

Everything I did became a challenge. It took me longer to get ready for work because I couldn't decide what to wear, or I couldn't remember where I put things. I was jittery, anxious. My hair had started to thin out and so did my body. None of my clothes fit; they hung off my shoulders. The woman staring back in the mirror didn't look good.

Sixteen days after the first chemo, I started to lose the muscle mass I had so painstakingly built over many years at the gym. My triceps and biceps were disappearing, making way for soft, undefined arms. My hips became so narrow, I could touch my hip bones. My breasts had started shrinking too.

I began to notice the color of my skin shifting to cancer gray. I had to adjust the color of the foundation and rouge on my cheeks. I found eyelashes stuck on the mascara wand and saw my eyebrows thinning.

Looking good was going to take so much more effort! I was willing to put in the work to go under the studio lights and in front of the cameras. I needed the normalcy of doing the work I had loved for decades, and I wasn't going to let breast cancer take it from me.

I zipped up a polka-dotted sleeveless dress, slipped into a pair of black heels, grabbed my makeup bag, and headed to work. The usual 8-minute drive to work felt longer. Concentrating on the road and traffic was more of a challenge as I traveled south on Mesa street toward 4140 Rio Bravo. I pulled into the KVIA parking lot and sat in the car for a few minutes, trying to gather my thoughts and strength to begin the day.

I opened the door and accidentally dropped my purse, which spilled everything onto the pavement. The tube of lipstick rolled underneath the car. My phone fell face down, cracking the screen!

"Damn it!" I cursed to myself as I quickly gathered everything and stuffed it back in the purse. I was in a hurry because the editorial meeting was starting in one minute. If I were late, I could be locked out and not allowed to participate. With my purse in one hand, and my makeup bag in the other, I pulled open the first glass door of KVIA, scrambling the best I could to get in!

As I opened up the second door, I noticed a lot of people were crowding the lobby. For a brief moment, I worried that I had forgotten some important event or guest coming into the studio. Scanning the lobby, I realized that some of my coworkers were gathered there, and they were wearing pink wigs and pink dresses. There was pink everywhere!

KVIA receptionist Debi Wilson took the items off my hands, grabbed me by my arm, and led me to the "step-and-repeat"[1] the station had made in my honor. Pink paper flowers in all shapes and sizes framed the words "Stand with Estela." It was a labor of love from my coworkers in sales and the traffic department, who carefully cut the paper flowers and glued them one by one onto the canvas. To the left was a dessert table, full of towers of pink cupcakes, strawberry flavored with whole strawberries in the middles and pink cream icing swirls on top. Glass beverage dispensers held pink lemonade, and other tall containers were filled with pink and fluffy cotton candy.

There were pink M&M's scattered atop the pink shimmering silk tablecloths and chocolate wrapped kisses in pink foil and

---

[1] A "Step and Repeat" is a display, usually with the same logo printed all over it, where interviews can be conducted, or pictures taken. It gets that name from how such displays are usually used, like on a red carpet at the Oscars. People "step" and have their picture taken, and the next person "repeats."

square mints, all in shades of light pink! The setup included pink yogurt-covered pretzels and pink cups and plates.

As I took it all in, I felt the blessings being showered over me, and I thanked God I worked where I did. My work family at KVIA put on their pink armor to help me fight this war.

CHAPTER EIGHTEEN

Las Picosas

Picosa means spicy in Spanish. It's also the name of a women's cycling club at Her Gym. I was part of the spicy ladies team up until I received my diagnosis. Before that, I was spinning three days a week! I stopped because I knew I had to use my energy to fight my breast cancer. I knew my immune system would be compromised, and I couldn't afford to expose myself to any germs that would take advantage of that.

That's the thing about cancer. It's not just the cancer cells that are a danger. Once you start chemo, even something as small as getting a cold can make you so sick you need to be hospitalized. Even a cold can be deadly. Cancer is a whole new level of fight.

I'd also stopped going to the gym because I didn't want the Picosas to feel sorry for me. I didn't want them to notice my hair and weight loss. The fight with my stupid pride kept me away from a group of strong and determined women who are serious about cycling.

Before things had gotten serious, I was signed up to ride twenty-five miles in the Chile Pepper Challenge, a run that brings in money for the El Paso Humane Society. After beginning treatment, I didn't have the stamina to participate in the grueling challenge, but I still wanted to show my support. Wearing my red Picosas shirt, I headed out to surprise them in the parking lot of Grace Gardens in El Paso's upper valley.

It was a cool and crisp September morning, and the parking lot was filling up quickly with cyclists and spectators like me. I watched the participants unload their bikes and secure their helmets and sunglasses under the bright sun. Some sprayed sun block and mosquito repellent and made sure they had enough water to make it through the ride.

"Estela, great to see you! We're riding in your honor. We wanted to show our support for you and all the other Picosas facing a cancer diagnosis," said Lety Jimenez as she put together pink ribbons to pin on everyone's shoulder.

I've known Lety for several years. She'd been with me, Paulina Scott, and another friend, Lory, for a five-day cycling tour in Oregon. I fell and broke three ribs on that cycling tour, and Lety never let me give up or feel bad about it. She's a go-getter who inspires everyone around her. Lety organized the team to participate, and she rallied the Picosas to raise awareness about breast cancer with a pink booth.

The Picosas hugged me, and we all teared up. It was a beautiful gesture of camaraderie and sisterhood. We posed for pictures and used our hands to make a shape of a heart as a sign of love and hope.

"Thank you, gracias, for remembering me and other women on a breast cancer journey. I appreciate you," I said as they made their way to the starting line.

If I had let my pride dictate what I was going to do, I would have missed this. Following my heart, instead of my pride, was a choice and an important lesson. The journey of cancer, like most things in life, isn't something we have to do alone. God will put people in front of us to help if we let ourselves accept that.

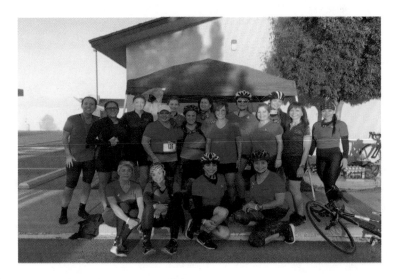

CHAPTER NINETEEN

The Cloistered Nuns

Tucked away in an unassuming neighborhood in Mesilla, New Mexico is a monastery. The grounds are surrounded by a pecan orchard where the Discalced Carmelite Nuns of Las Cruces live and pray. A longtime friend of Jimmy's who finds refuge and peace in this sacred place knew we both needed some spiritual strength to get through the journey. We set aside a couple of hours one Saturday morning and made the 40-minute drive from El Paso.

Weeks before, Diana had given me a brown scapular she bought at the monastery. Diana told me: "Wear it around your neck and only take it off when you shower. Make sure you place it near the cancerous tumors growing inside your chest." Along with the scapular was a note that read: "Take this scapular. Whosoever dies wearing it shall not suffer eternal fire. It shall be a sign of salvation, a protection in danger and pledge of peace." I was wearing the scapular under my dress and strategically placed inside the bra cups.

Diana De Lara-Zamudio is the general manager of Univision, the Spanish language station in El Paso and a devout Catholic. "I believe the two of you need some spiritual healing and guidance. I know Sister Trinidad will help bring strength and peace in the journey ahead," Diana said in a quiet voice as we pulled into the monastery.

Jimmy got out of this truck and we locked eyes through the windshield and half-way smiled. We were both feeling a little apprehensive but arrived with an open heart and open mind. Jimmy held my hand as we walked inside the small shop. Jimmy grew up in the Presbyterian Church but didn't undergo a formal religious education. He was way out of his element but was there to show support and find anything to help me get physically, emotionally, and spiritually stronger.

As we made our way inside, I noticed the wrought-iron wall that splits the room in half. It felt almost like a jail. We found it strange and a bit divisive at first, but learned the enclosure is a safe space where the Carmelitas live away from the hurried and sinful world. Cloistered nuns take a vow of self-denial and austerity and spend their days praying in silent contemplation. The Discalced Carmelites dedicate themselves to a life of prayer. Their roots are traced back to the 13th century in Mount Carmel in the Holy Land.

The room was quiet as we browsed through sparse items on the shelves. Religious icons, rosaries, small bags of pecans, and even organic honey are for sale. We signed in and rang the bell. A nun wearing a long, brown habit greeted us: "Buenas tardes.

Como estan? Good afternoon. How are you doing?" Sister Trinidad de Dios wore a white veil around her face and neck. Her cheeks were rosy, her eyes sparkled, and her smile was sincere and joyful. Sister Trinidad de Dios's presence exuded peace.

She quickly put us at ease when she said: "Les vamos a cantar para darles la bienvenida! We want to sing to you to welcome you to our home!"

A couple more nuns entered the enclosure, pulled out their music sheets, and began singing. Tears started rolling down my cheeks feeling overwhelmed as the Holy Spirit enveloped me. Both Jimmy and Diana's eyes welled with tears and smiled at the special dedication.

It was God's grace that led us to this spiritual and magical place. Sister Trinidad de Dios pulled me to a corner of the room and began praying. Her voice got softer as she leaned into me and said: "Tu eres una mujer de amor. Dios te ha regalado la gracia de amar incondicionalmente. Entregas tu corazón a todos los que te rodean. Representas amor! El mundo necesita mas personas como tu! El tiene muchos planes para ti, para que hagas el bien. You are a woman of love. God has gifted you with the ability to love unconditionally. You give your heart to everyone around you. The world needs more people like you! He has plans for you to meaningful things," she said.

Her words shocked me as I listened and tried to comprehend. Sister Trinidad de Dios's faith and words of hope and encouragement quickly calmed my anxiety and apprehension. It felt like she was delivering a message from God. Then suddenly she said: "Le vamos a ofrecer una misa para que Dios la sane. Vamos a la capilla para orar," she added. "We want to offer a mass for God's healing. Let's go to the chapel to pray," she said.

I was in a daze, still trying to decipher her words. With some wet and dry tissues in hand, we made our way outside to the small chapel a few steps from the enclosed quarters. The chapel smelled of incense and fresh flowers. There too was a wrought-iron enclosure, except this one was white, fancy, and elaborate with swirls. Behind the altar and five niches with icons and at the center Christ on the cross. Sister Trinidad opened the gate and led me to the statue of Our Lady of Mount Carmel to offer a prayer. She is the patroness of the Carmelite order and wears a crown of twelve stars that represent the twelve tribes of Israel and the twelve apostles. Both Jimmy and Diana stood behind the enclosure.

As I stood in front of Our Lady of Mount Carmel, I silently asked her to intervene and ask God to erase the cancer inside both breasts. I felt a chill and a deep sense of peace, as if she had agreed to my prayer and request.

The nuns held mass and sang, sounding like a choir of angels. We left the monastery spiritually charged. Jimmy may not have understood the conversations in Spanish but he felt the energy. Diana felt satisfied she had accomplished her goal. All three created a special bond that filled out hearts with reassurance that love, faith, and hope are the things that get us through any challenge in life, including cancer.

CHAPTER TWENTY

Fight with Me!

Inspiration is *everywhere*.

Case in point:

Jimmy Dick, my BMAC, is a hugely successful and savvy businessman. He is president and owner of the Viva Auto Group with 17 dealerships in El Paso, Las Cruces, Albuquerque, and Santa Fe. The Dick family has been in business in El Paso since 1904, with ventures in Mountain Pass Canning, Old El Paso Mexican Food, and Carter Vending. Jimmy purchased the old Courtesy Chevrolet on Montana Ave., and he reopened it as Ole Chevrolet. It's now Viva Chevrolet. He knows a thing or two about sales; it's in his veins.

Jimmy and I were on a plane to Sausalito, California, thirty thousand feet in the air, when we came up with a new way to raise awareness and money for the Stand with Estela fund. He had already helped me lay the groundwork for the fund itself when we teamed up with the El Paso Community Foundation.

We tossed around some ideas and strategies, and we finally came up with the "Fight with Me" slogan and campaign. He was always one for action behind his words, and within a matter of days, Jimmy and his team had two dozen service vehicles wrapped in pink and white with the Fight with Me logo. Strength, Courage, and Hope marked one side of the vehicles. On the other sides, just this: Fight like A Girl.

His marketing team ordered thousands of pink bracelets with #standwithestela embossed in white. There were hundreds of cardboard license plates and black license frames, also with the #standwithestela logo.

The promotional campaign included life-size cutouts of me in a pink cocktail dress and pink boxing gloves. The marketing team set up a green screen in Jimmy's office, making for a fun photo shoot to capture the images!

"Flex your biceps!" said photographer Heber Gandara. Click, went the shutter release. "Give me a jab and hook!" Click. "Let's try an uppercut and a cross. Hold it." Click. Click.

The Fight with Me campaign rolled out a week later. We distributed bracelets, displayed the life-size cutouts, placed pink ribbons outside the dealerships, and hung pink balloons inside for the kickoff event.

On a cool September morning, Jimmy and I went to all the dealerships to share my story and encourage employees to get invested in the campaign. Our first stop was the Viva Nissan Store. All the employees, from sales to parts to admin, gathered around me to listen to me tell of my journey and how Jimmy was a big part of it.

"Good morning, I'm Estela Casas, and I am fighting breast cancer. Today we are kicking off a campaign to raise awareness and money for the Stand with Estela fund to help women with gift cards or a wig, like the one I'm wearing." Thousands of dollars from the fund had already been donated to the Rio Grande Cancer Foundation to distribute in gift cards. At the Hospitals of Providence we had donated dozens of special undergarments with side pockets that hold the drains following a mastectomy to women leaving the hospital.

This was personal, but it was about to get even more.

"You just know Jimmy as your boss, but I want to tell you a little something about him. He has sat with me through chemo and held my hand throughout the process. He encourages me to fight to win this battle, and that's why we came up with the Fight with Me campaign. Jimmy is a kind man who lifts me up to fight every day. Will you join in the fight?"

Everyone at the store cheered.

"Take care of the women in your life . . . your mother, wife, sisters, aunts, grandmothers, friend, girlfriend, coworkers, and neighbors," I added, as I shared some of the challenges facing me, my family, my friends, and my community.

The support we were seeking was clear in the people I spoke to. Some wore pink shirts; all were sporting a bracelet, and most were moved by my testimony. They began asking questions. I answered honestly. It wasn't hard to see or understand; everyone is touched by cancer.

The Viva Dodge, Chrysler, Jeep store was decorated with pink balloons and the team greeted us wearing pink shirts and pink dresses when we arrived there. Everyone at the store formed a circle around Jimmy and me, and then they bowed their heads in prayer before I shared my testimony and asked them to believe in the campaign.

Our mission to rally the troops culminated at Viva Chevrolet, where we held a news conference. Reporters from broadcast and print media, from English and Spanish stations and newspapers, were there to support the Fight with Me campaign.

I was emotionally drained and physically exhausted, but the day was a fruitful, community-building one. Four weeks later, in October, each dealership came in with a check for the Stand with Estela fund. They'd raised $20,000, but most importantly, they'd raised awareness for something bigger than just selling cars, bracelets, and license plate frames. The funds would be used to distribute more $250 gift cards for treatment co-pays and incidentals. I received receipts from women who used the money to buy medication or vitamins. Some used it to pay for gasoline!

I'll always be thankful for the hundreds of Viva Auto Group employees who showed up, willing to fight with us.

CHAPTER TWENTY-ONE

Come Holy Spirit!

When your corazón and mind are open, your soul is ripe for transformation. This journey taught me many things about myself. I embraced my strengths and weaknesses, and I learned to accept, and ask for, help. I've allowed myself to be vulnerable.

I have also become more prayerful. I don't go to mass every Sunday, even though in my faith tradition, one is expected to do so. Mass is considered a sacred event, an opportunity to praise God. I consider myself a spiritual person, and I do praise Him in my daily prayers and through my interactions with others. As a spiritual person, I believe my grateful heart is what gets me through this tough journey, not just with cancer, but with life.

My open spirit has drawn people to me. Some tell me they include me in their prayers, others included me in their intentions during mass, and I met others who asked if they could pray over me for healing. I believe healing, in one way or another, was exactly what I experienced.

Just three days after my second chemotherapy treatment, Jimmy took me to the church he likes to attend. He is also a spiritual searcher. He feeds his faith when he learns more about the Bible, and he listens to the Pastor's message.

We arrived at Calvary Chapel Sun City on a warm, sunny Sunday morning in October. We made our way through the parking lot, holding hands, and we were greeted at the door with big smiles, firm handshakes, and warm hugs.

"Good morning, Estela. Good morning, Jimmy. Welcome to our church, enjoy the service!" said the greeters at the door.

I felt safe and comfortable, and I felt open to receive God's word and blessings. We made our way to the left side of the chapel. Jimmy held my hand, his big warm hand enveloping my cold, thin, frail one. Little did I know that God's healing hands would also touch me deeply that fall morning.

We sang. We cried. We listened. We learned.

Pastor Terry Grey talked about how words can give life or destroy life. Proverbs 18:21 (New King James Version) says, "The tongue has the power of life and death, and those who love it will eat its fruit."

As a journalist, I know the value of words. I am aware of using the appropriate words to tell a story more effectively. But that morning, I wasn't a journalist. I was just one of many in the congregation, longing to hear a message that would resonate in my heart and soul, that I could share and apply in my life.

I sat quietly, absorbing every word and listening intently to the sermon. I thought of all the people I was that day: a woman, broken from a failed marriage of thirty-two years, a mother of two adult children and a teenager, a sister whose siblings are far away, a member of a community that cares for me deeply, a friend, a lover, and a cancer patient fighting the biggest battle of her life.

I recalled the times that perhaps I didn't choose my words wisely, blurting something I didn't mean to say. I thought back on all those times I intentionally offended someone I loved. Words that are spoken in anger can never be taken back, even with a heartfelt apology. My heart felt suddenly heavy with guilt, shame, and regret.

In silence, inside my heavy heart, I asked God for forgiveness. As Pastor Grey asked the congregation if we were ready to receive the Holy Spirit and be healed, I felt he was speaking directly to me. I began feeling light-headed, and I broke into a cold sweat. My hands were balmy, and droplets started forming on my forehead.

Jimmy felt my hands and asked, "Are you okay?"

"I don't feel well. I need some fresh air," I responded.

I felt the walls and tall, pitched ceiling closing in on me. I couldn't see straight, and I thought I was going to faint.

"I need to go to the restroom. I don't feel well at all," I whispered in his ear. Jimmy helped me up and led me out. The congregation was praying, but I felt their eyes follow us out.

Jimmy led me to the entrance of the women's restroom and stood outside. I stood in front of the mirror and splashed my pale face with water. I didn't recognize the woman staring back at me. My eyes were glassy, the color in my cheeks was gone. Something had changed inside of me, and it was manifesting itself on the outside.

Jimmy noticed too when I walked out. He looked terrified, teary-eyed, and pale. I recall stepping down the couple of steps toward the parking lot, but I can't remember the rest. Jimmy held my arm tightly so I wouldn't fall.

I faintly heard a woman's voice say, "Estela, can we pray for you?"

I remember stopping and nodding "yes" because I was unable to speak. Jimmy held on to my arm, and another woman held me up as my body went limp. I couldn't breathe. I had trouble focusing my vision, but I could sense a bright light enveloping me. I chose to surrender to it.

The woman held me and prayed over me. She kept saying, "Lord remove the cancer from her body." The other woman prayed, too, but I didn't understand the words. She wasn't speaking in English or Spanish. In a daze, I realized she was speaking in tongues. God was speaking through her, a powerful and transformative moment in the mundane middle of the church parking lot.

I believe it was the Holy Spirit speaking to me inside the chapel, through those faith-filled women. It was both terrifying and comforting.

After a few minutes, I opened my eyes, and everything was soft and bright. I recall seeing the women's faces, but I don't think I could pick them out in a crowd. They were so fuzzy. Everything around me was beautiful. The Franklin Mountains looked more majestic, the sun was warm, and the sky was bluer than it had seemed when we walked into the church.

I was surrounded by love, prayer, and healing words and hands. I prayed in silence, *Come Holy Spirit, get me, my family, and those who love me, through the journey with grace and dignity.*

He listened.

The Holy Spirit touched my soul!

CHAPTER TWENTY-TWO

Merde!

My digestive system has always given me problems. That's why proper nutrition has always been an important part of my life. After years of painful and embarrassing episodes, I discovered I was lactose intolerant. Ice cream, milk, and cheese were put on a list of foods to not eat.

I had read that chemo would wreak havoc on my appetite and digestion. Chemo, always up for a challenge, did not back down for me. All the discomfort and embarrassment I'd experienced from lactose intolerance returned with a sickening vengeance. Only this time, it was *everything* I ate. The little I could stomach, mostly chicken and vegetable soup, came out of my stomach and intestines violently and unexpectedly.

I forced myself to drink a lot of water, even though water tasted terrible to me. I had to stay hydrated if I didn't want to wind up in the hospital. I drank almost a gallon of water a day to help flush my body of the toxic drugs.

Around the ten-day mark following a treatment, my intestines would start churning in my body. Uncontrollable diarrhea followed. Most people (including me!) don't like to share their bathroom habits, but I am, because it's important for you to know if you're about to embark on a cancer journey. It's important that those around you know too.

I had several episodes where I just couldn't control the outcome. Most days I was at home, and I could handle accidents in the hallway or near the bathroom. I had to throw away several pieces of clothing. My body was getting rid of medication that destroyed the good and bad bacteria in my gastrointestinal tract. It was all indescribably disgusting.

I was determined, however, to remain active during chemo. One day, I decided to go out for some exercise and a little "retail therapy" at the outlet mall in Canutillo. I had dropped about ten pounds and wanted something new to wear. I slipped on some yoga pants, a shirt, and tennis shoes. I wrapped a cotton paisley handkerchief around my bald head and threw on a baseball cap and big sunglasses.

"Good morning, can I help you find something special?" asked a young lady at the Michael Kors store.

"Good morning. I'm just browsing, thank you," I answered as I made my way to the sales rack in a back corner of the store. I was looking for brightly colored clothes to help lift my spirits and help brighten the cancer gray of my skin.

There were more employees there than customers that

morning, so I had the store mostly to myself. I browsed while the sales ladies arranged the high-end purses. I could feel them staring at my wrapped head.

I had found a pretty yellow blouse, and I got in front of the mirror, holding it up to imagine how it would look on me. Yellow has always been a good color for me, and I liked the look of the blouse. Suddenly, my intestines started making unusual noises, twisting and turning in my cancer-flattened belly. It felt like I had a baby inside doing somersaults. And like a little one misbehaving, the twenty-five feet of intestines didn't care that I was in a public place, or that I was by myself. They didn't care that I was in a store with strangers.

And right there, next to all the pretty blouses and skirts (*All items up to 50% off!*), everything came gushing out. There wasn't anything I could do to stop it, and I was horrified. I froze and squeezed my butt cheeks, hoping I could make my way to the employee bathroom. "*God, please get me to the restroom!*" I begged in silence.

A young and beautiful sales lady noticed what was happening and came to my rescue. She saw me shaking and unable to move, and she lovingly took my shaking arm, and led me to the bathroom on the other side of the store. She brought paper towels to wipe the mess I had left in between the sales rack and the midi dresses.

"Don't worry about it. I just want to make sure you're okay," she said with tears in her eyes.

"I'm so sorry," I said in a trembling voice.

"No worries, I'll get you some clothes to change into," she said as she led me inside the bathroom and closed the door.

I looked down at my soiled pants, and I felt tears beginning to well up in my eyes. I leaned on the door, sobbing as I pulled off my tennis shoes, socks, and pants. I threw everything inside a black plastic bag I found in the employee bathroom while the young lady stood outside. I used up the entire roll of paper towels and toilet paper to wipe myself up.

Outside the door I heard: "What size jeans can I bring you?"

"Please bring me a size 6 and a medium-sized shirt. I was looking at the yellow one on the sales rack," I responded in between sobs.

She brought me a size 6 and a size 4 skinny jeans. I can't recall the last time I fit into a size 4! I washed my face, adjusted the scarf on my head, and the new outfit on my body, and opened the door. She smiled and led me to the cash register.

"Thank you so much for your help. You've been very kind. I'm sorry," I said as I handed her my credit card.

God, please get me out of here! I said to myself, hoping no one else had noticed.

I will be forever thankful to that young lady. She was an angel, helping a stranger in need. I have a feeling her life changed that day. Mine certainly did. Realizing how vulnerable and fragile I had become was sobering. I made myself a promise that day: from that point on, I would listen to my body before my ego. That "retail therapy" cost both of us way too much.

CHAPTER TWENTY-THREE

Stelhita, Scarlett, and Daniela

Auburn. Platinum blond(e). Highlights. Lowlights. Silver.

All these choices can be found inside three by five boxes at your neighborhood Walgreens or CVS for about twelve dollars. They all promise to "cover up the gray," to make your hair shiny and supple. Women have so many options on how to wear our hair. I've had it permed, straightened, shoulder length, but mostly short. You never really appreciate your hair—even if it's thinning or gray—until you lose it.

Nineteen days after the first chemo treatment, my hair started to fall out. Strands of hair detached from my scalp. They appeared on my shoulders and fell on my breasts. They fell on the floor, leaving behind a trail. Thin, delicate reminders of the journey I had just begun, one hair at a time. I squeezed a pea-size amount of shampoo on my head, hoping not to disturb the follicles. I thought that if I gently rubbed my scalp, the hair would not fall off so easily.

I was wrong.

In the shower, I felt chunks of hair lathered in shampoo slither down my body to my feet and down the drain. Seeing my hair covering the drain was sobering. Picking it up with a tissue was too. Naked, wet, and terrified, I stood in front of the mirror holding a tissue with my hair and wondered what was next.

What was next?

A hairstorm!

As I began to dry it to get ready for work, the storm began. Hairs flew all over my bathroom, being pushed by the hot air of the blow dryer. They landed on the gray and white speckled granite countertop. More were on the cream-colored tile below. I quickly swept the hair with my hands and tossed it in the trash can.

I had known I would lose my hair, but I was totally unprepared for how gut wrenching it would be to ACTUALLY lose it. I had to find solutions, take action, and stop pretending that I didn't need a wig just yet. I opened the closet drawer and gently pulled out a white box. Inside was a beautiful brown wig I had ordered online.

Weeks before, Sandra and Toni had taken me shopping for wigs. I tried on a pink pixie, a blue and black bob, and one that looked like my own hair cut. We brought home all three. I told myself,

One is for work, and the other two are for fun.

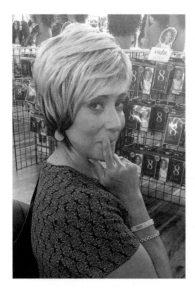 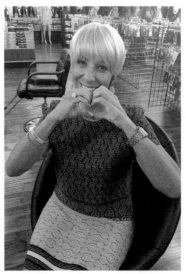

And leave it up to my kids to find humor in everything! They picked out names for the three wigs, and I wrote them on the plastic head mannequins. "Stelhita" was my work wig because it resembled my hair color and cut, but unlike my real hair, the chestnut color of the synthetic hair was shiny. She was there for everyday use, but her debut was anything but.

It was October 6th. That morning, I was going to have my second chemotherapy treatment. Later in the afternoon, I was to get a prestigious award from the University of Texas at El Paso. I got Stelhita out, combed her, placed her on the mannequin, and placed her in the passenger side of my car. I wrapped my head in a pink handkerchief and threw on a pink baseball cap, and then I headed to the infusion center for the 7-hour treatment.

Fernando was with me, carrying my "chemo bag" full of treats and water. I also got a special visit from Erika Castillo of KFOX and her husband, Shawn. I had just settled into my recliner when they arrived with gifts. Erika brought me a fuzzy gray blanket to keep me warm and a pink frog stuffed animal to make me smile.

Mas pequeños milagros.

I was anxious to get through the treatment, hoping the chemo would drip into my IV faster.

"Can we speed it up? I have a speaking engagement at UTEP. I was named a Gold Nugget, and I will be delivering a speech," I asked the nurse as I pointed to the machine.

"No, Ms. Casas, we can't. We have to space out the drugs every ninety minutes," she answered with a smile.

"I brought a change of clothes, so I'll change here," I added.

I had to be at the Stan and Lee Rubin center for the news conference KVIA-TV had set up to make the announcement after I was chosen as the 2017 outstanding alumni from the College of Liberal Arts. I became a Gold Nugget 12 years after I earned my degree in Broadcast and 35 years after I first enrolled at UTEP. I was being recognized as an advocate of women's and children's health issues.

I kept a close watch on the fluid in the IV, and I had already slipped on my black heels and skirt. Once the nurse unplugged me from the machine, I ran into the bathroom, shrugged into my suit, applied some makeup, sprayed some perfume, and put on Stelhita. I rushed out of the center toward my car and put the pedal to the metal.

The Rubin Center was packed with well-wishers. Some people I didn't even know were there to congratulate me and thank me for my contributions. Familiar, old self-doubts crept in as I listened. I wondered about the contributions I have made to UTEP. I'm just a journalist who has been reporting the news for thirty-six years in my community.

After an introduction by the Dean of Liberal Arts, I got behind the podium and delivered my prepared speech, thanking everyone, and trying to accept the Gold Nugget Award, graciously, without letting doubts or fears make me stumble. I looked at my brother in the audience, listening intently to his little sister. He had never heard me speak in public before. I think I made him proud. Sandra, who was also recognized as a Gold Nugget, was sitting in the first row. The College of Health Sciences picked Sandra because of her work in the community. She is also an adjunct physical therapy professor at UTEP and mentor to dozens of students. Jimmy was there too. I acknowledged their presence and smiled, but I looked just above their heads to speak and avoid distractions. I knew that if I looked into their eyes, I wouldn't be able to get through my words of gratitude. My heart was pounding, but I pushed through the range of emotions, tempered by the drugs circulating through my body. A university photographer snapped some pictures with UTEP President Dr. Diana Natalicio and other university administrators. Everything was kind of a whirlwind.

My brother and Sandra whisked me away when they noticed I was running out of steam. I went home and took a power nap to prepare for the next activity at the president's residence. Dr. Natalicio was opening her home for a dinner party that night to honor the Gold Nuggets and distinguished alumni.

Jimmy rang the doorbell, looking dapper in a navy-blue suit and trademark lavender shirt, tie, and paisley silk handkerchief. His shoes were black and shiny, and he looked dashing with his deep dimples and sheepish smile!

I'd pulled a different wig for the evening too; it was a cute little number that was longer than Stelhita and cost thirty dollars. My children had chosen a name for her too—Scarlett Overkill from *Despicable Me*—because it was sassy and sexy. I *felt* sassy and sexy in my black fitted dress and five-inch stilettos, even after seven hours of chemo, even with Scarlett on my head, secured with two-sided tape. Daniela (the pink pixie) would come out another day.

But that day? That day, Stelhita and Scarlett did just fine, and so did I.

CHAPTER TWENTY-FOUR

Katy Berry

I got a call one afternoon from Catherine Berry, a counselor from Ascarate Elementary. She told me her students had raised money for the Stand with Estela fund. Her school was the first to get behind the cause!

I excitedly agreed to be there November on 1st, to cap off Breast Cancer Awareness month and accept the donation. I made the 20-minute drive to Ascarate, which is located on Alameda, south of the freeway. It's near the refinery, surrounded by used car lots. The old campus sits protected behind a wrought iron fence.

I'd dressed up for this very special occasion, including securing Scarlett firmly to my head with double-sided tape. By this point, I had already lost all of my hair, but I had a bounce in my step, thinking gratefully how amazing it was that at this campus, these students were pitching in to help the fund.

Katy greeted me when I arrived, wearing a big smile and a pink shirt with a picture of the school mascot: the Ascarate Eagles. We hit it off immediately. She quickly led me to the library, which was decorated all in pink.

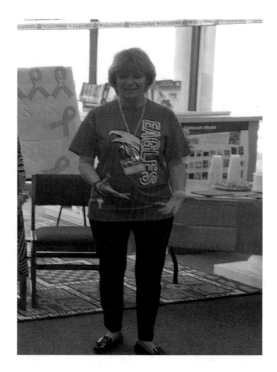

The sun was shining brightly through the tall windows. It was a terrific backdrop for a big pink poster with pink ribbons that spelled, "Welcome Estela Casas with Stand with Estela."

The teachers, staff, and even some of the children also wore pink ribbons and shirts to mark the special occasion. The principal, Mrs. Claudia Ureno-Olivas, and several other teachers greeted me with firm handshakes and warm smiles.

Katy put together a beautiful table with pink mums and green grapes to share with the children. She introduced me to them and told me how they'd raised more than $700 for the fund. Those precious kiddos beamed with pride in themselves, and in their community. A camera from the Ysleta school district was recording the presentation. Students (reporters-in-the-making!) were taking notes and writing down questions they wanted to ask in one-on-one interviews.

I thanked them for raising that money. Then I turned and hugged Katy, grateful for her efforts and her example. The kids and I talked about what to do when confronted with challenges. It was a very personal sharing moment for me, but also for them. They, too, raised their hands and shared.

Just three days later, I learned that Katy had been tragically killed in an all-terrain vehicle accident. I was devastated.

Katy was my age. She was out with her boyfriend on an ATV, having fun. I've done that a few times. She had found love. I had found love again too. But now she was gone, and I was four treatments into my fight to stay alive.

Although I had just met Katy, I felt connected to her, and her generous heart. I had seen the difference she made in her community, just by being who she was, and doing what she did best: teaching. I resolved to carry her spirit with me, thankful for our brief, but powerful, encounter.

I wasn't the only one.

Ascarate elementary students and teachers continue to donate to the Stand with Estela fund.

They do it because Katy taught them well.

They do it in her honor. They do it because Katy loved, and they love too.

CHAPTER TWENTY-FIVE

Cancer High

During my high school years, drinking alcohol wasn't a big deal. Like so many of us in the Borderland, I'd cross the bridge to Ciudad Juarez on the weekends to dance at the Electric Q and drink a few Cuba Libres, rum and coke with a splash of lime. The legal drinking age in Mexico is 18, but I looked older. I got away with ordering a drink or two at a discotheque at 17 and even 16! It was the cool thing to do, especially since I felt there was nothing cool about me in high school. I was a homely and nerdy choir girl.

But everybody I knew went to Juarez to party! I couldn't party hard because I had to be home at eleven. My parents knew I would go to Juarez with my high school sweetheart. Arnoldo got me home at eleven o'clock sharp, safe and sound. My breath smelled of peppermint chewing gum and a little alcohol.

Despite these little adventures, I never really drank a lot, and I never experimented with drugs. It wasn't because I didn't have the opportunity. Truth be told, fear was my motivating factor. I was too afraid my parents and older brothers would find out, and they wouldn't trust me anymore.

A few days after I shared the news of my diagnosis with family and friends, I got a visit from my godson. He came bearing gifts, not with beautiful wrapping paper or elaborate bows, but in brown paper bags. We hadn't seen each other in years, but we always reached out during important times in our lives: graduations, confirmations, weddings, and funerals. This visit was because cancer had crept its way into our lives, and he wanted to help me on the journey.

"Hi Nina!" he said with a big smile as I opened the front door. He is effusively affectionate, and he gave me a warm and reassuring hug. "I brought you a little something you may need down the road," he said with a mischievous grin.

"Thank you!" I said, happy to see him. "Let's open it in the kitchen."

In the kitchen, I placed the brown paper bags on the counter.

"What's this?" I asked as I pulled out several packets.

The small ones read: "Sativa Medi-Drops," with a warning at the bottom: KEEP OUT OF REACH OF CHILDREN. On the back, nutritional facts in bold letters: Sugars 11 grams, Carbohydrate 17 grams, 70 Calories. In smaller print: Medical Cannabis (10 pieces) 10 mg THC.

"Medical marijuana? For me?" I asked, bewildered at this gift.

"It's all for you, just in case you need it," he said.

My godson had meticulously and lovingly written descriptions for what was in there. Indica was described as "sleeper" to help me relax, sleep, and relieve the pain. The other was labeled sativa as the "upper," just in case I needed a boost of energy, or if I needed help with the loss of appetite during chemo. There were lollipops in different flavors and Medi-Drops. The larger bags contained sugar cookies. Every item was packing 10 milligrams of THC!

I sifted through the cache of medical cannabis and nervously asked, "You want me to get high during chemo?"

He answered with a question. "Why not?" He added, "This isn't for recreational use. You may have severe nausea, or anxiety, and taking a Medi-Drop once in a while will help you get through the process."

It made sense. Cancer patients sometimes need medical marijuana to help numb the physical and emotional pain of fighting cancer. There I was, standing in my kitchen with bags of medical marijuana that's illegal in Texas! The drops, cookies, and lollipops had tetrahydrocannabinol, which, in higher doses, is classified as a hallucinogenic drug. Did I mention it's illegal in Texas?

"Thank you. I appreciate your gift, but I have to put it away in a safe place, under lock and key. Remember, Andres is only thirteen years old," I said as I nervously scooped all the packets and quickly stuffed them in the bags, along with the instructions.

"Promise me, Nina, you'll take a Medi-Drop or eat a cookie if you feel nauseated or you're losing too much weight," he said.

"I promise—but ingesting medical marijuana will be a last resort. I wouldn't want to be drug tested and have Dr. Valilis ask me why THC showed up in my blood work!" I answered, only half joking.

We both smiled and made a pinky promise. We didn't dwell on cannabis. On his way out, he gave me another tight hug of reassurance, knowing he had done his part in helping me navigate through the challenge ahead.

"Love you, Nina," he said, with his heart in his voice. "Please take care and let me know how it goes. If you need more, just give me a call."

"I will," I answered, fearing I might indeed need cannabis to help me navigate through.

Later that night, alone in my bedroom, I looked through the sugar cookies, Medi-Drops, and lollipops again. I placed them all in a closet drawer. I was nervous about breaking the law, but I felt grateful for my godson's thoughtfulness. In my heart, I hoped I would never feel nauseated enough, or be in so much pain, that I would resort to popping a Medi-Drop in my mouth or chewing a special cookie.

But that day did arrive. It was four days after the fourth chemo when the nausea got to me. I could barely stomach chicken soup, and even water tasted awful! I was at home alone and decided to take a Medi-Drop. I was shaking when I broke open the paper baggie and popped a pink tablet the size of a quarter in my mouth. It dissolved about thirty minutes later.

The Medi-Drop tasted funny and left an aftertaste in my mouth. It tasted like hope. Within another thirty minutes, the nausea went away. I felt more relaxed and less guilty about "getting high." I remembered a quote by poet John Lyly in his 1579 novel,

Euphues: The Anatomy of Wit: "All is fair in love and war."

I was no longer worried about breaking the law. My godson's love was helping me with my own war with breast cancer.

CHAPTER TWENTY-SIX

Jardin de la Esperanza

Flowers make me happy and fill my heart. Despite my humiliating experience while shopping, I decided to shop again, but this time, for my garden of hope.

I used to have beautiful roses, but we pulled them out to pour cement to make room for a basketball court. I had transplanted a few red, white, and pink geraniums and Calla lilies to some larger pots on the back porch. The roots had outgrown the plastic containers and needed more space to continue growing. I wanted roses again.

I headed to Home Depot. Everything is green and blooming there in spring, and the aisles are lined with pink, red, white, lavender, and yellow roses, including every shade in between.

I loaded the cart with one in every color, and I even picked up a few annuals and perennials that were on sale. I squeezed seventeen plants in the cart, several bags of Miracle Gro, and some gardening gloves. Nutritious soil, appropriate watering, sun, and some TLC is what makes for beautiful gardens (and people too). I walked out of the nursery excited and full of energy. My son had already dug the holes, and I had to till the soil with mulch and the compost.

I asked one of the associates to help me get all the lovely plants inside my car. The friendly man with the orange-colored apron was about to line the trunk with plastic sheets when he recognized me.

"Are you the lady on the news? You're Estela Casas, right?" he asked.

I looked down at his name tag and answered, "Yes, Mr. Hernandez. I am. I'm starting a gardening project at home."

"I so admire you for sharing your story. You are a brave and courageous example to other women. You give everyone hope. Can I give you a hug?" he asked.

"Of course—and thank you for watching!" I answered as he gave me a hug. I never turn down hugs, especially when they are offered with good intentions.

I watched Mr. Hernandez carefully place plastic on top of the car mats and arrange the plastic pots. He had a friendly smile and long salt-and-pepper hair. Although his long locks blew over his face in the morning breeze, I could see his eyes were glassy with tears. His voice got shaky as he asked, "How are you feeling?"

"I'm blessed, and I'm actually feeling well enough to start a big gardening project," I answered.

"I'm so glad, Ms. Casas. My wife and I include you in our prayers," he added.

"Thank you," I said humbly, my heart moved by his kindness.

Moments like these made sharing my battle publicly worth it. I question sometimes if sharing so much could be detrimental to my well-being, and to the well-being of my family and my relationships. But hearing how my journey touched that man's heart answered that question.

Sharing has helped me stay focused. It is actually cathartic being able to express my feelings openly. I did several news stories to chronicle my journey, but I know there were times when I didn't have to say anything. People could see the transformation I went through on their TV set at home. They, like Mr. Hernandez, noticed my clothes fitting loosely, the wigs, my painted on eyebrows, and my glassy eyes with droopy fake eyelashes. The chemo made my eyes water, and the glue on the fake lashes caused an allergic reaction.

All of those transformations only emphasized to me that life is precious. The beautiful plants in my trunk were a reminder of the circle that is life. I hoped that the roses would blossom for decades and that I'd get to see the roses bloom in the fall. I hoped that the roots of perennials, the purple salvia, and the pink peonies would grow deep enough through the winter and flower in the spring, and that begonias and dahlias produced a few times before their circle closed and they died. On my way home, I wondered if I, much like my new plants, was in the middle or near the end of the circle. And did it matter?

I, too, was growing, in spite of—maybe even because of— my cancer. New opportunities to bloom were all around me. Mi Jardin de la Esperanza was the perfect place to reflect that, and to remind me every day to keep on going.

CHAPTER TWENTY-SEVEN

Squirrels!

I know a little about a lot of things and not a lot about anything. Many people can recite scripture and poems or remember dates in history, but not me. Lack of attention or lack of interest? Perhaps a little of both.

Even before I experienced the effects of "chemo brain," my memory had always been squirrelly. The first time I noticed the fuzzy little creatures inside my brain wreaking havoc on my memory and ability to retain information, was after the birth of each of my three children. Lack of sleep and nursing didn't help. I recall sitting in a rocking chair in the middle of the night nursing my three babies as they emptied my breasts of fresh milk. I would stare into their innocent eyes, lost in them. Nursing is a huge commitment, but so rewarding when your baby looks up and smiles between gulps and lullabies I would sing in English and Spanish.

Oops!

See?

Squirrel!

During my bout with thyroid cancer in 2010, the squirrels came rushing into my head. Carolina was 21, Marcos was 16, and Andres was 7 years old when I was diagnosed with thyroid cancer. The thyroid is part of the endocrine system and is a vital organ that regulates the body's metabolism. I had brain fog and emotional ups and downs. One hour I was feeling fine, and the next I was crying, feeling super sensitive, and easily offended. I'll blame it on the hormones. Women suffering from an underactive or overactive thyroid are easily misdiagnosed as having depression. Then I discovered the lump in my throat and was diagnosed with thyroid cancer, and everything made sense. The diagnosis gave me a reason and excuse for my seemingly odd behavior. There was a real reason the squirrels were running in my head. I have a vivid imagination, and I pictured the squirrels on an exercise wheel inside a cage going round and round and round. With a diagnosis and treatment, I was able to attack the problem, and the medication helped tame the squirrels in my head.

During chemotherapy to treat my breast cancer, they appeared again. Except this time, the mischievous squirrels stole words from my mouth. There were times when I couldn't find the right words. I couldn't remember people's names. I wasn't thinking straight, and I couldn't put together a thought to communicate properly. Luckily, I had a teleprompter to read at work, but every-day conversation was a huge challenge because the squirrels ran away with my words and held them like a delicacy. I've learned to switch back and forth between English and Spanish when I can't remember a word, but suddenly that wasn't working either.

I felt dumb, embarrassed to hold a conversation. I found myself stuttering and stopping mid-sentence to search and find the appropriate word. I stared a lot as my brain tried to process.

There. Goes. A. Squirrel!

Chemo brain is for the birds!

Do squirrels like birds?

Squirrel!

A real squirrel, not the ones swirling around my brain, ruined the flower bed in the front yard during my chemotherapy treatment. She was smart, fat, and mischievous! I think she had to be a female because she outsmarted everyone in my house. She, and proba-bly her mate and babies, nibbled through all the leaves and roots of the plants that once thrived in the flower bed next to our front door. Every geranium, rose bush, bougainvillea, ranunculus, and forget-me-not was gone, along with the roots! The squirrels dug deep holes, creating an elaborate maze under my house, active and obviously entertained with the delicacies!

We set out a trap with peanut butter to entice her taste buds. Not a single squirrel took the bait. We poured cement down the hole, but they dug one next to it. I was told that sprinkling red chile powder would discourage them, but no luck there either. I gave up and pulled out the dry plants and scooped up the soil; after that, I brought in new compost and didn't plant anything. The family of squirrels moved on because there wasn't any food left to eat.

The squirrels in my head are still there. There is plenty of food for them to snack on. I've learned to acknowledge them and the role they play in my brain. I think it's actually what keeps me active and engaged at home and at work. I, too, search for that acorn, berry, or root to keep me pushing forward. I'm just glad they haven't been back to burrow in my flower bed, although I sometimes see one run across the front yard.

CHAPTER TWENTY-EIGHT

Failure Is Not an Option

The morning after I received my diagnosis, I didn't even think of Plan B, or opening up door number two or three. I had no alternate plan. I've done so many stories on early detection month after month, year after year, and repeated the phrases on live television:

"Early detection saves lives."

"Cancer doesn't have to be a death sentence."

Looking back, deep down, I wasn't sure about the truth behind those words, although I delivered them with conviction. I wanted to believe. After I found out I had cancer, I had to believe them. I had no choice but to believe them. The tumor on my right breast was bigger than a sweet pea. It was technically considered stage one, but it was a higher grade and was aggressive, kind of like me: chiquita pero picosa—small but spicy.

I didn't catch it early. The mammogram I had 8 months before didn't catch it, either. Between December and August, the cancerous tumor grew into a 1.6-millimeter mass deep in my chest. The mass on the left breast was 2 millimeters and had a tiny mass on top of it. My 2 breasts had worked in harmony to feed 2 tumors at once. It's known as synchronous formation. It's rare, and accounts for only 2 percent of newly diagnosed breast cancers. Early enough? Only time will tell. Cancer isn't always a death sentence, at least at the beginning it isn't. That's when one has the most energy and will to live, fight, and get through the process.

Six months into the journey, I still never considered the possibility that the chemotherapy wouldn't kill the cancerous tumors inside my breasts. I told my oncologist, Dr. Valilis, that I'd turned into the poster child/woman for breast cancer, and I was afraid that I was giving people false hope.

He said, "Estela, some women never develop cancer and die of something else. The cancer returns in other women a year later. Some women die in the process because the cancer is so aggressive and resistant to chemotherapy. Don't feel like you are giving false hope. You are brave to share your story and educate your viewers about fighting cancer every day. Keep doing what you do and share your journey. You're helping a lot of women and families. It's not false hope. It's understanding of the journey."

Perhaps I was naive about sharing my personal side of battling breast cancer. Perhaps, unlike me, others fighting this ruthless disease had a Plan B, C, and D. My Plan A was to fight hard and with faith. I turned it all over to God. I had a team of family, friends, and doctors, and I had a community that lifted me in prayer and surrounded me with love, encouragement, and positive vibes. They would not have allowed Plan B to enter my head, much less my heart.

Faith continues to carry me through the dark moments when I realize what my family and I have been through. I never doubted we would successfully get through all six rounds of chemotherapy. It never crossed my mind that my body would reject the toxic, but necessary, poison running through my body.

Chemo is a fucking bitch, and everybody experiences its effects differently. It wipes out the bad *and* the good cells in your body; and yet, I never doubted it would work in mine.

I've said before that cancer is a mind game, and it's true. I prayed and envisioned the chemo-cocktail entering my bloodstream and eating away at the cells. It's tough to outsmart cancer because it can mutate, but it is administered in cycles, every twenty-one days. That's when the cancer cells are most vulnerable to an attack. The three-week interval allows the body to recover from all the damage caused by the previous treatment. The first three days I would feel okay, but days four through nineteen were tough. I couldn't eat and had stomach problems. A few days before the next chemo, I would actually feel quite normal before the next punch in the gut. The cycles were grueling.

I kept my attention on the strength of my body and the

strength of my faith. I turned to my God and my children and family to help me trust that we didn't need to consider a Plan B.

CHAPTER TWENTY-NINE

Chicken Pot Pie

Comfort food.

It's a meal that makes you remember your mom's chiles relle-nos or your grandmother's cinnamon and anise tamales. Chicken pot pie is not on my list of comfort food. I enjoy a medium Lomo Argentino and asparagus from Garufa, an Argentinian restaurant on Mesa street, or some bacon-wrapped scallops from Pelican's with a Vina Cobos Bramare Malbec. That's my comfort food!

One exception is cooking for others! Making a meal from scratch and sharing it with my family . . . now *that* makes my heart happy! As a Hispanic woman, and first generation El Pasoan, I am proud of my heritage, language, culture, and food. I'm not talking about enchiladas, tacos, rice, and beans. That's not real Mexican cuisine, even though those foods are tasty. Chiles en Nogada, cochinita pibil, pescado zarandeado, pollo en mole, escamoles, and chapulines, are just a few delicacies that make Mexican cuisine world-class. Escamoles are ant larvae and chapulines are grasshoppers and they are both delicious!

Cooking for others is one way I show love. I enjoy being in the kitchen making green chicken pozole, caldillo, and rajas con crema. The common ingredient is green chile from Hatch that I freeze after the harvest in September. I typically roast and freeze more than one hundred pounds a year! Making these dishes keeps me connected to my roots and connected to my loved ones.

I didn't cook much during chemotherapy, and my love for food faded dramatically. My taste buds died along with the good and bad cells in my body. I wasn't nauseated all the time; I was simply not interested in food. Besides that, everything I ate had a metallic taste, like I was chewing on a thin slice of steel. Even water tasted bad, but I forced myself to drink it to flush out the chemo circulating through my body. I forced myself to drink alkaline water, coconut water, and lemon water. None of them helped. I even gave up my morning coffee because the smell and thought of it turned my stomach. Salty foods were too salty, and sweets were too sweet.

Eating was no longer something I took pleasure in, but something I had to do. I needed to maintain nutrition, but the only thing I could regularly keep down was chicken soup with vegetables. Sometimes, I would only have the clear broth because the taste and texture of the chicken made me want to vomit.

During this time, I received several gifts of food from friends who wanted to save me time in the kitchen. My friend, Angie Rosales, ordered me specially prepared meals. Estrella Escobar and her two girls, Mia and Estrellita, delivered Italian food, and Martha Aguayo made her famous chicken soup. El Paso's First Lady, Adair Margo, even lovingly prepared a chicken pot pie she thought might tempt my taste buds! After all, she told me, it is *her* comfort food, a recipe from her grandmother. It was a beautiful round pie filled with creamy vegetables and chunky pieces of chicken, and golden brown with scalloped edges. Piping hot, it smelled delicious!

I was humbled knowing that she shared this dish, made from a recipe passed down through generations of her family, just for me. I forced myself to have a spoonful as I imagined all the love and blessings in that chicken pot pie. As I chewed a piece of chicken covered in cream sauce, I closed my eyes and listed my ingredients for this recipe:

4 cups of prayers

4 cups of well-wishes

4 heaping tablespoons of hope

4 heaping tablespoons of encouragement

Sprinkle of humor

I was able to eat only a couple of tablespoons, but my boys cut out big slices and scooped them onto their plates. I felt peaceful, watching how they enjoyed the pie cooked with loving hands and good intentions. It was a delicious reminder that a bit of comfort can go a long way toward filling our bellies and nourishing our souls. That chicken pot pie did both that day, for me and for my sons.

CHAPTER THIRTY

Virgen Peregrina

A year before my diagnosis, a special visitor began living in my home. The icon of the Virgen de Guadalupe, the patron saint of Mexico, arrived in a 2x16-inch cardboard box, by way of my neighbor, Delfina.

"Buenas tardes, Estela, como estas? Habla tu vecina Delfina Barriot. Tengo a la Virgen Peregrina de la Familia. Te gustaria tenerla en tu casa?" she asked. ("Hello, Estela. How are you? This is your neighbor Delfina down the street. I have a traveling Virgin. Would you like to welcome her into your home?")

I answered, "Si claro que si." ("Yes, of course.")

I really didn't know what she was talking about, but I agreed. Delfina delivered the box. Inside, there was a gold-colored wooden box with a cross carved on the outside. I carefully pulled it out and opened the two flaps at the same time. In the middle was a picture of the Virgen Morena, also known as Mary, cupping her hands in prayer wearing a green robe with stars. On the right side was a small white sack holding a wooden rosary, along with instructions on how to pray with it. On the left was the Ideario, the ideology or mission of the traveling Virgin: to encourage praying the rosary every day as a family. It's an international Catholic Movement, the Movimiento Regum Christi, and its goal is to promote the Catholic faith. Its motto is to "Love Christ, Serve People, and Build the Church."

The Holy Rosary is a prayer that uses beads to recall four mysteries or events in the lives of Jesus and Mary: Luminous, Joyful, Sorrowful, and Glorious. The prayers of the rosary include The Lord's Prayer and the Hail Mary. Catholics believe this prayer of repetition and meditation is important to protect against all evil. The inscription at the bottom of the box is a prayer dedicated to the Virgen de Guadalupe, who Saint John Paul the second described as the Mother of the Americas.[1]

I set up a small shrine in my living room along with a candle. I welcomed her into my home, but not in my heart. During that

---

[1] Patrons believe the Virgen de Guadalupe appeared to Indian Juan Diego four times on the Tepeyac Hill in Mexico City in 1531. It is said that she instructed him to ask the bishop to build a chapel in her honor. When Juan Diego told the bishop the story, he didn't believe it, and he asked Juan Diego for proof of the holy visit on the hill. During the fourth apparition, she asked him to gather some flowers. He obliged and filled his mantle with flowers and delivered them to the bishop. When he dropped them on the floor before the bishop, an imprint of her image appeared on his mantle. The bishop built a church, and in 1976, a basilica was built around the shroud. Millions of pilgrims visit the site every day to pay homage. More information: www.pilgrimqueen.org

time, I was praying the Mary Untier of Knots Novenas, and I did not pray to the Virgen Morena to intercede on my behalf, to calm the unrest and instability in my home and life.

I pray every day to God. He and I have a relationship. Sometimes, He speaks to me in subtle ways, and other times, He sends very loud and life-altering messages. He has done that several times. I consider myself a spiritual and faith-filled woman, always searching for God's grace and mercy. I don't go to church every Sunday, but I strive to be an honorable and good person. Every day, I make the conscious effort to ask myself, *How will I make a difference today?* It's a self-imposed challenge.

Just three families in the neighborhood participated, so the Pilgrim Virgen de Guadalupe came back to my home every three months. The month I was diagnosed, she was not in my home. That quickly changed when my Delfina heard the news.

"Estela, ahorita te llevo a la Virgensita para que rese por ti y te sane," Delfina reminded me when she called. ("Estela, I'm dropping off the Virgin so she can pray for you and heal you.")

When la Virgen returned, instead of taking up her spot again in the living room, she found her way to my bedroom, where she still watches over me. She's surrounded by pictures of my family, and I often pray the rosary to ask her to intercede on my behalf for healing, and to keep my children safe and healthy. She's a calming force when I am feeling anxious. Her eyes, gazing lovingly downward, and her tranquil face, with skin the color of mine, bring peace to my heart. The Virgen Peregrina remains in my home after Delfina died suddenly, while I was undergoing treatment.

CHAPTER THIRTY-ONE

Ring the Bell!

The morning of December 28, 2017, dawned at a crisp 40 degrees, to my full and grateful heart. My children, Carolina, Marcos, and Andres, had all been home to celebrate a beautiful Christmas, and that day was going to bring even more cause for hope and celebration.

December 28, 2017, marked the last of 6 chemotherapy treatments.

We prepared a breakfast feast with eggs and chorizo, homemade salsa, flour tortillas, and sautéed red potatoes with onions. I skipped coffee but had a slice of toast and picked at the eggs. I was already too nervous and excited.

My dear Sandra had given me a new custom shirt for each of the first five chemo treatments, but that day's shirt was the most special of all. The shirt was black with long sleeves and pink lettering, and it read, "Last Chemo 12/28/17." I also wore the black and pink tennis shoes she ordered with my name on the back, black workout pants, and pink socks. Sandra had single-handedly turned me into a cancer fighter fashionista.

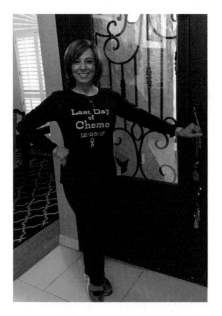

I dabbed on some makeup, giving my cheeks a rosy glow that said, "Screw you, cancer!" despite my pale and puffy face. I had trouble gluing on my eyelashes because I didn't have any more real eyelashes to hold the fake ones up. My eyes kept watering. I had big hair from Scarlett that made my shoulders look small and my body shrunken. I had dropped twenty pounds.

None of that mattered. Today was my last day of chemo.

The kids and I got in the car and drove off with the radio blaring. We sang and danced in our seats all the way to the infusion center. None of them had ever been inside the center or seen my chemotherapy infusions. Work and school got in the way.

Nothing got in the way for my dear friend Sandra. She was with me during all six chemotherapy treatments because she didn't want me to be alone.

I saw the excitement in their eyes, knowing we were about to clear a big hurdle. Carolina, Marcos, and Andres had all been beaten down emotionally and physically. The strain of the unknown weighed heavily on them too. They, too, had lost weight and suffered sleepless nights. The struggle manifested itself in all of us, body and soul.

We had never talked about what those four months were really like for each of us. Instead, we observed each other in silence, looking for—and following—unspoken cues.

And still, all of that paled against the fact that we were together at that very moment, fighting and gaining strength from each other. No one wanted this treatment to succeed more than my daughter and two sons.

"We're here!" I said, yelling above the music in the car. They all stared at the signage. Their bodies stopped dancing and their voices went silent. Carolina, sitting in the passenger seat, smiled. In the rear-view mirror, I observed my sons' eyes open wide. All three looked uneasy, but they were determined to face the day. They were understandably apprehensive about what they were about to experience.

We got out of the car, carrying a bag full of snacks and water bottles for the long day ahead. The glass doors of the center opened, and the receptionists greeted people in the waiting room with a warm smile and a friendly "Good morning!"

"Good morning, Ms. Casas; you can go right in. This is your last chemo treatment! You have a lot to celebrate," the receptionist said.

"Yes, I brought my children to help me ring the bell," I said excitedly.

"It's going to be a good day," she answered.

"Yes, it is!" I called back as we headed past the hall to the elevator.

"Good morning," I said to the nurses at their station, waving as we passed several patients with their feet propped up in recliners, IVs running.

"This is my favorite spot," I told the kids. "This is where I can see everyone coming in."

I sat down, pulled the right lever to raise my legs, covered my legs with a blanket, and settled in. Their eyes revealed their apprehension, so I tried to make them feel more comfortable, using my smile and positive attitude.

"Good morning, Ms. Casas! Today is your last treatment, and you get to ring the bell," the nurse said with a smile.

She had wheeled in the cart with the bags of medication that I would be administered for the last time. She showed me the names of the drugs, to make sure I knew what was going into my veins.

"You know the drill," she said as she opened the sterile alcohol wipes to clean the port-a-cath. Carolina was sitting next to me, holding her breath, as the nurse instructed, "Take a deep breath," inserting the special needle.

Carolina cringed, but she didn't say anything.

"It's in. Here are your two Tylenol caplets and water for your last treatment," she added.

"Yes, thank God. This time, I don't want the stuff that makes me drowsy," I responded. I normally got an anti-anxiety pill before treatment to help me relax, doze off, and get through the seven-hour infusion.

Only two people were allowed in the infusion room with each patient, so the kids took turns checking up on me. As I sat quietly with my feet propped up, I quietly observed them all.

Carolina had flown in, taking time off from her new job in Dallas. She's a beautiful, strong-willed, no-nonsense young woman who is well spoken. She didn't say much that day, but her eyes expressed hope.

"Do you have enough water? Remember, you need to drink a lot of water. Can I bring you something to eat? Are you warm enough?" Carolina asked as she made sure the pink blanket covered my legs.

"I'm fine; thank you Mami," I answered. Why do I call her Mami? It's tradition.

Carolina would smile when she caught me looking at her. She has dimples and almond-shaped brown eyes, and I thought, *How lovely she looks today, with less worry and more hope.*

I am blessed to have such an amazing young woman as a daughter. I wondered what she thought of me, and the way I chose to go public with my journey, becoming vulnerable and exposing us to criticism. She never intervened or questioned why I chose to share my most intimate details. She understood the purpose and goal.

I thought, not for the first time (or last), about the effect of all of this on my children. We all aspire to be admired by our children, and we hope to leave them a legacy they can be proud of. I want Carolina to remember me as a strong woman who had the courage to get uncomfortable enough to continue growing through my own pain and the biggest challenge in my life. A failed marriage had already beaten me down. I wasn't about to allow cancer to break me. Instead it molded me into a better version of myself. I believe she saw that on this day.

"I'll sit here with Mom, now," said Marcos as he traded places with Carolina. "How are you feeling, Mom?" he asked.

"I'm good, Papi," I answered.

Marcos has hazel-colored eyes with thick eyelashes. He looks like my dad. He has a happy disposition, but this journey had drained him and changed him. I looked deep into his eyes to try to get a sense of how he was feeling. Marcos also looked at me with hopeful eyes. I smiled at him and dozed off for a few minutes.

When I awoke from my power nap, Andres was sitting next to me, his beautiful dark brown eyes tearing up. At age 14, he had the toughest time comprehending the gravity of the situation. He was just a few months away from getting his braces, and he was going through the awkwardness of being a teenager in middle school. I felt a real rush of compassion for him, as he had to navigate not only those things, but also his parents' separation and divorce, and my cancer diagnosis, all in just eighteen months. My baby was growing up fast, under pressure.

I had been afraid to observe my children up to this point. I'd actually avoided being more keenly aware of their actions and emotions. It was a protective mechanism. I felt it was my responsibility to lift them, not the other way around. I guarded their hearts, by guarding mine. I knew they were suffering, and knew of their sleepless nights, but I didn't show them mine.

A parade of people started coming in to help us celebrate!

"Hi, guys!" Sandra said, holding a bouquet of pink heart-shaped balloons.

One balloon read, "Celebrate Courage." Another spelled out "Congrats" in bold letters. The balloons were attached to a bouquet of beautiful pink roses, white hydrangeas, and a soft pink ribbon.

"Hey, Sandra," we all answered as she went down the row, hugging everyone. Sandra has a heart of gold, and she's a positive force in all of our lives. She's a friend, mentor, and lifeline. I love her like a sister, and my children love her as an aunt.

My childhood friend Griselda, and thyroid cancer sister, Nicole, also spent the morning celebrating with us. Toni came too, with her big smile and big personality.

All of these friendships are . . . pequeños milagros . . . bendiciones.

A coworker and photojournalist from KVIA walked in with a camera and tripod in hand to record my last chemo. He'd set up and started recording when the nurse removed the IV from the port-a-cath and inserted the Neulasta right above my hip. Neulasta is an expensive, but effective, drug that makes the body produce white blood cells to avoid infection. I never got sick from a secondary infection during treatment, and my immune system was never compromised.

At around 3:00 p.m., it was time to close the chapter on this part of the journey. Emotions ran high, and tears started flowing as the nurses led us to the hallway and the celebratory Bell Wall. My friends formed a circle of love around me and my children.

"You have successfully completed six rounds of chemotherapy.

You are brave and courageous, and the nursing staff and everyone at Texas Oncology wish you the best," said the nurse as she handed me a certificate of completion. Then she added, "Before you ring the bell, read the inscription to your friends and family."

Holding the certificate in my hand, I began reading the phrase: "Ring this bell three times well to celebrate this day. This course is run, my treatment done, and I am on my way."

I reached up, grabbed the cord, and rang the bell three times, marking the end, and giving thanks to God for the strength to complete the course with courage, determination, grace, and dignity.

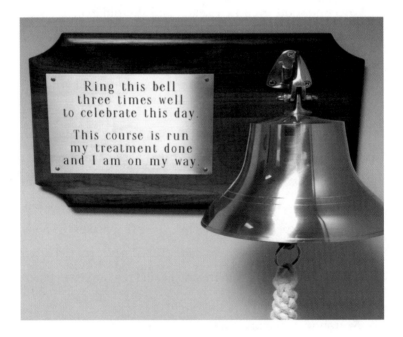

CHAPTER THIRTY-TWO

Los Colores of Cancer

The cancer journey has been painted in a rainbow of colors. Red represents cancers of the blood. Light blue signifies prostate cancer, and white represents lung cancer.

I wear a pink bracelet, engraved with #standwithestela. It's a two-toned plastic bracelet that reminds me of the daily challenges and struggles faced not only by me, but by the thousands of women and their families on this painful journey. The Rio Grande Cancer Foundation ordered hundreds of them to distribute when we created the Stand with Estela fund.

Pink is the color of hope and everything pretty. I love pink, fragrant roses, peonies, carnations. I like wearing pink outfits and lipstick because I believe it's a flattering color on my skin. After my cancer journey, pink represents my survival, and new beginnings too.

Cancer made me aware of all the color of life around me. The colors that make the sunsets and sunrises in El Paso's Upper Valley and New Mexico became even more breathtaking. The reds and oranges native to west Texas are spectacular! It's not that I never noticed them before, but now they looked even more breathtaking.

When I was diagnosed with breast cancer, I believe I became more connected to my humanity. I felt more vulnerable, facing my mortality. Yet, in some ways, it was like being born all over again. In that new alive-ness, my eyes and heart saw and felt all the wonderful things around me I didn't see before, and everything in it looked more beautiful. I observed the trees and flowers blooming, and now I saw them complete their circle of life.

I know there's a scientific explanation for the different colors in the sky, and why clouds form, but I choose to believe it's God's work to make us pause, inhale, admire, and be grateful for His greatness every time we look up to the heavens. It's a shame I needed a cancer diagnosis to notice and acknowledge God's hand is in *everything*! He is the one who gives us the gift of sight to see all the beauty that surrounds us and the capacity to feel.

That February, before the surgery that would remove my breasts, I traveled to Cancún, Quintana Roo, Mexico, with Jimmy. He had a working trip in Mexico and invited me to join him, his son, his daughter-in-law, and his top employee. We stayed at a resort on Punta Cancún, where the waves of the Gulf of Mexico and the waves of the Caribbean crash, meet, and mingle.

We stayed in the Turquoise Tower at the Hotel Ziva in the adults-only section and enjoyed a spectacular view. Our suite was on the third floor, facing the crystal clear water. One early morning, when Jimmy went downstairs for a meeting, I made time to be alone with my thoughts. I stood on the balcony and watched the sun rise above the blue waters of the Caribbean. I stood in awe of nature's beauty and took in several deep breaths. My lungs filled with the salty sea breeze and the mist covered my face and bald head as I attempted to understand its beauty and power.

I felt as small and insignificant as a grain of sand, tossed in that turquoise water. Listening to the waves crashing, swirling, I closed my eyes for a few minutes and held on to the glass fencing, imagining life under that water, visualizing the coral and different colored fish swimming beneath the sea foam and white water. I've been snorkeling before; but this time I didn't want anyone to see my bald head.

Time stood still as I imagined the water and clouds in a dance choreographed by nature. Forceful yet graceful, the waves crashed against the natural rocks and man-made barrier that protect the beach and grandiose hotels. The views are free. The Mexican constitution says all its beaches are accessible to anyone. It is federal property, and everyone has the right to enjoy the beach, a piece of heaven. I heard people laughing, and I spotted a couple with two young children setting up a blanket. The mother carried a grocery bag. She set it down and dug her feet in the sand, watching her husband and kids play in the water. Seeing the young family enjoy the water and time together, I couldn't help but smile. The mother handed her family towels to dry off, and they gathered to have burritos for breakfast. The simplicity of it all filled my heart with joy.

They savored the burritos and Coca-Colas, and that little slice of heaven had the children squealing and giggling under the morning sun. They hugged their mom and dad saying "gracias," thankful for finding that magical spot on the beach!

I wondered if they noticed the shades of water gradually shift from baby blue to turquoise green to deep navy. I wondered if they noticed the double rainbow on the horizon.

Cancer changes the way we look at color and the world around us.

Cancer. Changes. Everything.

CHAPTER THIRTY-THREE

Hearts on Our Sleeves

Cancer encouraged me to celebrate everything, especially the gift of another day.

The infusion center at Texas Oncology looked especially bright and festive that February. Red and pink hearts dangled from the ceiling, celebrating the month of love and friendship. With renewed love in my life, and my heart filled with promise and joy, the Valentine's theme was a welcome one for me.

The noise from the TVs was low, but I could still hear the chatter. Beeping sounds from the IV machines signaled when to switch out the meds. A week before February 14th, there was more activity than usual. No one wanted to be hooked up to an IV on that special day. The nurses were busy with patients. I noticed new smells from the fragrant perfumes and colognes the men and women sprayed on that morning. Love was in the air!

My normal recliner in the corner was taken, but I felt compelled to find another spot, as if something were directing my steps toward another side of the room. I would only be there for 90 minutes, so I decided to explore and let my feet do the walking. The chemotherapy treatments, which had lasted 6 to 9 hours, had transitioned into 90-minute infusions of Herceptin, an immunotherapy drug I was administered every 21 days.

Herceptin is a targeted treatment for HER2- positive cancers. According to the American Cancer Society, Herceptin attaches to HER2 receptors to fight tumor growth. Researchers believe the adjuvant therapy stops the cancer cells from growing and dividing, and it may actually signal the body's immune system to destroy that cancer cell. It's promising therapy for the second most aggressive cancer. I could only hope that was what it was doing in my body.

God directed my steps to a recliner near two women. I was going into work later that day and had to be "camera-ready," so I was sporting a new wig and wearing a gray and pink polka-dotted dress. I sat down, lifted the lever, and admired my sexy five-inch gray heels and legs on the faux leather chair. The outside reflected the way I felt inside: sassy, confident, and hopeful. It was quite a different look from previous visits, when I was administered the chemo and didn't have to go back to work.

My eyes scanned the room, saying hello with a smile, as I settled into my chair. I observed a woman, perhaps in her thirties, sitting to my left, alone. She wore a long black wig. Her eyes seemed glassy and looked weighed down by the long eyelashes framing them. She squirmed, looking uncomfortable with herself, with the environment.

I guessed I probably looked like that, too, during treatment. Sitting in one place for six to seven hours is a challenge! The big leather chair seemed to swallow her small, fragile body. The black pants she was wearing hung on her narrow hips and thin legs. Her green bomber jacket was loose-fitting around her shoulders, draping down her thin arms to veiny hands.

She caught me looking at her, and I smiled. She smiled back, seeming to welcome the moment. Her friendly disposition belied the sunken appearance and dullness of her eyes. I didn't know what kind of cancer she was fighting, and the reporter in me knew I couldn't ask. I wasn't a reporter at that moment anyway. I was just another woman fighting cancer, sharing feelings of despair, strength, and hope.

Right across from me was another woman hooked up to an IV. The contrast between her and the woman to my left was striking. For one thing, her disposition was very different because she wasn't by herself. Her husband sat on a chair next to her, and he lovingly held her hand in his. She wasn't wearing a wig. Her bald head was wrapped in a black scarf. The paleness of her face accentuated the dark circles under her eyes. She didn't have eyebrows or eyelashes around her eyes, and there was sadness and despair in them.

I observed how the two of them interacted as a couple. I could feel their anxiousness as the chemo cocktail dripped into the port-a-cath in her chest. They both looked exhausted.

Cancer does that to you, emotionally and physically.

She looked up and said, "Hi, Estela; how are you?"

"I'm doing okay," I responded as positively as I could. "How are you?"

"We're here again, doing this a second time around since the first treatment didn't work as planned. We're hoping the new chemo cocktail does the job," she answered.

"God is good. We have to have faith it will," I answered.

It occurred to me then that we three women, all in different circumstances, were sharing the same vibe that day. We were cancer patients hoping to become cancer survivors, and we were creating a bond. We became cancer sisters.

The phone in my purse began to vibrate, startling me from those thoughts. Dr. Valilis's name was flashing on the screen.

"Hi Estela, I have the results of the MRI," said Dr. Valilis.

Dr. Landeros had ordered a second MRI to compare the one I had when I was first diagnosed six months before. He needed to see how the tumors reacted to the chemotherapy before he performed the double mastectomy, just two weeks away. The hope was that they had gotten smaller or even disappeared.

"Did the chemo work?" I asked with hope in my heart.

Dr. Valilis answered immediately.

"Yes, the chemo shrunk the tumors. The tumor in the right breast shrunk from 1.6 centimeters to 5 millimeters. The tumor in the left breast, that had a smaller tumor on top of it, shrunk from 2 centimeters to 10 millimeters. The chemo ate away more than half the tumors! That is very good news, Estela."

"That's fantastic news, Dr. Valilis," I responded in a soft voice.

I didn't want anyone to hear me, especially knowing the two women next to me were still undergoing treatment, or in a second round of chemo.

"Yes, it is. I'll see you in two weeks, after the surgery," said Dr. Valilis.

I celebrated inside my heart. There are so many hurdles to clear and small victories to celebrate during a cancer journey. I had cleared a small one, but I quickly reminded myself the journey wasn't over. It would never be over, even if I were declared cancer free. With cancer, it's not a matter of if it will return, it's a matter of when.

I said a prayer, and as I looked up beyond the ceiling to thank God for the good news, I noticed the IV bag was empty. Herceptin was circulating in my body like a Pac-Man eating away at the cancerous cells. The nurse came over, pulled out the needle in the port-a-cath, and placed a bandage with Garfield the Cat over the injection site.

He made me smile.

CHAPTER THIRTY-FOUR

Respira Profundo, Be Grateful!

The body I didn't like was serving me more than I thought. Every cell, muscle, and fiber in my body had been flooded with poison during my battle with cancer, and *it was still working!* I became proud of my body and its strength. It took a room full of women in gym clothes to remind me that the body is a walking miracle.

My friend Toni held a fundraiser for the Stand with Estela fund at Pure Barre the night before surgery to remove my diseased breasts. My dear friends Patti, Toni, and Nicole wore yoga pants and tops, ready for the strength training and stretching class.

Pure Barre was abuzz with many ladies working their core. We quickly assembled in a room lined with mirrors. I wasn't participating because I needed my strength for the following morning, and I had lost my voice to laryngitis! I sat on the carpet and observed how they tilted their necks, outstretched their arms, placed their legs on the ballet bar, and pointed their toes. Their bodies seem to glide in slow movements, using their own weight to elongate their muscles. They looked beautiful. I admired their bodies, even as I had a rueful moment, knowing that their bodies had not betrayed them like mine had.

Stop it! I thought to myself. *You never want anyone to have to feel the way you have!*

My heart shifted from feelings of betrayal to feelings of gratefulness. I'd completed six rounds of chemo and nine of eighteen immunotherapy treatments. I was a few hours away from major surgery to remove both breasts, *and my body was still fighting!*

I let the music and choreography take me to a different place in my head. In that journey, I realized that even though my body was not as strong at that *moment*, it was actually serving me more than I thought.

Gazing into the mirror in front of me, I smiled and acknowledged that I was strong.

I was ready.

The instructor said, "Breathe in. Be grateful. Hold it. Be kind to yourself. Hold it. You're strong. Exhale through your mouth. Push through the diaphragm and empty your lungs of stress from work, the husband, and the kids. Let's do this a few times.

"Good job ladies, class is over. Thank you for helping raise money for the Stand with Estela fund, and thank you, Estela, for allowing us to help women in our community fighting breast cancer. We will be praying for a safe and successful surgery tomorrow. Sharing your journey so openly is inspirational and is a testament to the strength of your body. We are here today to build on that positivity you transmit to strengthen and honor our bodies."

I got up and whispered, "Thank you for helping make El Paso a better place to live."

As I drove home with a grateful and hopeful heart, I thought, *It was all of us, sharing that positive energy tonight.* I prayed that the blessing of that would carry on through my surgery the next day.

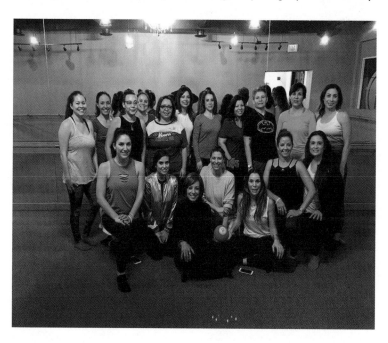

CHAPTER THIRTY-FIVE

El Roble
(The Oak Tree)

The distance was short, but it was still a long drive home. The final thing I needed to do before my surgery the next day was heavy in my mind. For six months, we had worked to get to this point, this moment of truth.

To close the chapter and open a new one on this journey, I wanted to shave off the little hair that had grown back.

Ten weeks after the last chemo, peach fuzz had sprouted on my head, with silver hairs that stood straight up like thin wires on my egg-shaped head. The hair was soft and fine; in between all the shiny platinum strands were dark brown curly hairs.

The coming day was yet another new start in my cancer journey. I was determined to begin the next chapter cleanly, with a shaved head. I pulled out the trimmer I had used for my boys in between haircuts. I handed it to my son, Marcos.

"Will you do the honors?" I asked.

With a serious look, Marcos answered, "I will, Mom."

"Start from the neck area and move up to the top of my head in even motions," I said with firm determination.

Marcos didn't say a word. He didn't have to. I could sense he wasn't happy about shaving his mom's head. He flipped on the switch to the trimmer, and the buzzing sound filled the kitchen. I felt it as the fuzz began falling on my bare shoulders. The hair was so thin it slipped through my fingers as I tried to gather enough to snap this picture.

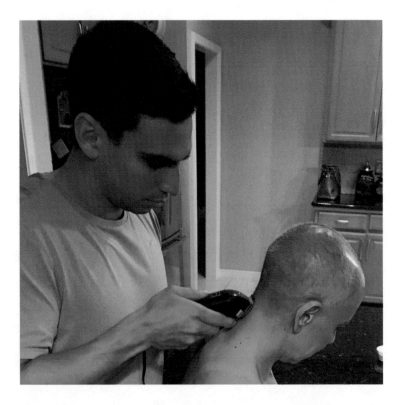

Buzz . . . Buzz . . . Buzz . . .

I focused on that sound and honored that moment with my middle son. I knew he wasn't exactly enjoying this task, but he understood.

For me, it was symbolic, a precious moment between us. We pruned the small branches of a diseased oak, making way for healthy growth. The oak tree is a life-affirming symbol of strength, resistance, and wisdom. My son's caring and love made me feel like a strong Roble that night.

"Thank you, Papi," I said emphatically.

Marcos smiled, kissed my soft head, and said, "You're welcome, Mom. Everything is going to go well tomorrow. Love you."

"Love you more. Goodnight," I replied.

I was ready.

CHAPTER THIRTY-SIX

Fuera, Cancer!

For such a highly anticipated day, Surgery Day arrived uneventfully. I got out of bed and opened the shutters to let the light in. The sun wasn't shining any differently. It was still bright and yellow, peeking through the cream-colored shutters in my bedroom. The clouds weren't any fluffier. Just a few white ones dotted the beautiful blue sky.

I showered with special antibacterial soap, disinfecting my torso. The rest of my body got its usual lathering of liquid Dove soap. It smells better than the hospital stuff! I stood in the shower, letting the warm water run down my breasts, which would soon be gone under my surgeon's knife. My eyes shed tears that swirled down the drain with the warm water. I quickly dried my body and slipped on a taupe-colored push-up bra and matching underwear from Victoria's Secret.

I had never needed a push-up bra before. In fifth grade, I went from a training bra to a "C" cup. I'd always had full breasts. I wanted to feel attractive and sexy under the button-down denim dress I'd bought specifically for that day. It wasn't anything special; I just had to make sure I could take it off easily. My breasts would soon be gone, and I would never again wear that same bra, or the dress. I wasn't going to need a push-up bra because my new breasts would be fuller and perky.

I slipped on some comfortable suede loafers to match the small gray designs on the denim dress. (I was a cancer fashionista even before surgery!) I applied a small amount of makeup I knew would be coming off; then I attempted to glue on some eyelashes. My hands were so shaky, I decided not to mess with them. Instead, I applied mascara on the short and scarce eyelashes that dotted my top and bottom lids and penciled in some eyebrows.

The nurses would have more important things to do than worry about my eyelashes! But they would be tasked with taking care of my wig. I was going to make sure everyone in the OR knew not to look under the wig and to keep it tucked in the surgical cap. I didn't want anyone to see my bald head. I even put extra double-sided tape to secure Stelhita.

My overnight bag was carefully packed the night before.

Makeup. Check.

Toothbrush, toothpaste, and deodorant. Check.

Eyelashes and glue to wear home. Check.

Extra underwear. Check.

I'd gotten up early on purpose, to set aside some time to pray for courage and peace. It was a short and casual conversation with God. His grace had carried me during the first part of the journey. I had faith He would carry me again. I felt at peace with my decision to have the double mastectomy. No hesitation. *Let's do this*, I told myself.

Jimmy drove up in his big truck. I opened the door before he even rang the doorbell, so happy to see him. We greeted each other with three kisses and nervous smiles. His dimples appeared smaller, and his gorgeous green eyes were not as bright. His smile was forced, his upper lip just a thin line. Jimmy wears his heart on his sleeve. I felt his heart beating faster, like it wanted to leap from his chest, as he attempted to hide his anxiousness. I embraced his emotions, but I couldn't allow his fear or doubt to overcome me. I put him at ease with my strength and faith, trusting everything would be okay.

He did look especially handsome that morning. My eyes drank in his six-foot-one frame, broad shoulders, and flat stomach. Jimmy wore his pressed button-down dress shirt, navy pants, and a thin leather belt with a silver buckle. He wore navy socks and shiny dress shoes. He smelled good, clean. Masculine.

I sighed, wishing we were going somewhere else together, and not to the hospital! It was a little chilly outside, so I pulled on a light coat, grabbed my bag, and carefully walked down the steep steps of my house to Jimmy's truck; our hands were intertwined the whole time.

I can't even remember what we talked about, driving down Mesa street to The Hospitals of Providence. I can't remember the traffic at eight thirty in the morning. I do know it was a lot of small talk because all the "big stuff" had already been said. There would be time for more of that later on. There were no adequate words to express what we were both feeling at that moment.

I remember focusing on his eyes, admiring his profile against the window. The eyelashes on his left eye curl up. The ones on the right eye curl down. I reached for his hand, caressed his fingers, and squeezed tightly. Just a touch to share my gratitude. My hand moved up his forearm toward his biceps, relishing the feel of his firm muscles. My strong and steady man! Before I knew it, we'd arrived at the hospital.

I was at peace, ready to move on to the next chapter. One deliberate step at a time, we made our way to pre-op, and we were escorted upstairs to outpatient surgery. We had the entire area to ourselves. I was asked to strip down and slip into the hospital gown and bright yellow socks. I could feel Jimmy's eyes on me as I changed. In a moment of mischief, I smiled and actually flashed him with my sexy push-up bra!

"You like?" I asked.

He smiled shyly, green eyes looking up from curly lashes, and answered, "I do."

The medical professionals began parading in. I could hear their steps behind the curtain. Soon they were parting the curtain to say good morning and begin asking questions.

My cousin Lety, who is also a nurse and a breast cancer survivor, came through the curtain. She had decided to take the day off to be with me. Lety knew the drill, personally and professionally. Diagnosed in 2008, she'd had several rounds of chemotherapy, a lumpectomy, and radiation. She's in remission. She brought me a sense of calm and good vibes.

Then my dear friend Nicole arrived. Next, my longtime friend Margie—who was at the hospital when my daughter Carolina was born, and was my labor coach when Marcos was born—also showed up. Other family members filed in, all letting me know I was not alone.

Our little corner of pre-op was getting crowded, so some family members were asked to go to the waiting room. Just knowing they were there, *somewhere*, made me feel happy and grateful. Their love and caring helped me remain calm. The drugs being pumped into the IV probably also had something to do with it!

I was wheeled into the radiology department for a nuclear test with an entourage in tow. Sentinel lymph node mapping helps determine if the cancer has spread to the lymph nodes near the armpits. I got four injections in each breast. The needle prick didn't hurt, but the isotope dye going into my breast caused excruciating pain as the liquid filled the lymph nodes. Lying on the gurney, with my breasts exposed, I could feel the hot liquid snaking through my chest. There's a short window of time to complete the test, so I was quickly wheeled into another room and propped onto the nuclear medicine diagnostic machine to try to find cancer in the lymph nodes.

"Hello, Ms. Casas; let's get you settled in. Do you need a blanket?" asked the technician.

"I'm okay, thank you," I responded.

"I'm going to go behind the plexiglass and give you instructions over the intercom. Try not to move. I'll tell you when we're finished," he said, all business and very reassuring.

Minutes later, he walked in, and said, "All done."

He helped me sit up, and then he moved me into a wheel-chair. We wheeled out past the friends and family in the waiting room. I smiled and gave them all a thumbs up, trying to soothe the forced smiles and worried looks on their faces. I pressed on, using my imagination to get me through the moment. I envisioned myself in a parade. I was the Grand Marshall, riding in a convertible, waving with one hand and holding the heavy crown on my head with the other!

The nurse took all of us to pre-op, where I had love and family around me again. I thought of my brothers and their wives, with me in spirit from Portland and San Antonio. My son Marcos arrived after his classes at UTEP. He sat with his eyes wide open, and it seemed like he wasn't even blinking. I could tell he was jittery. He didn't know what to say, so he just looked at everyone and smiled with gratitude. My thirteen-year-old son, Andres, was in school. Carolina was on her way to El Paso from Dallas.

Seeing my children suffer has been the toughest part of this journey. My heart has broken so many times, seeing how they've navigated through this process. They've seen me at my absolute worst, yet they would tell you it was my best, a display of courage and strength, pushing through the challenges.

Still, every time I had the chance, I would say, "I'm so very sorry." Both Carolina and Marcos responded, "Don't worry, Mom, we're okay." Andres, at thirteen years old, would declare, "We've already been through so much, anything that lies ahead will be a piece of cake!" Wise words from my teenager.

Certified Nurse Anesthetist Lee Hunt was about to pump Propofol into my IV and lead us in prayer. We all bowed our heads and held hands tightly in our circle of love, connected with God and with each other. You might not think it possible to find magic moments before this life-changing operation. I did, and it was that moment that I carried with me.

"I'll see you all in a few hours," I said as I got a hug and kiss from everyone, including Marcos's kiss on my head, and three kisses from Jimmy.

I looked down at my bright yellow socks with a smile. I grabbed my head, making sure my wig was secure and adjusted my hospital gown, ready for the trip to the OR.

I was still awake when I was lifted onto the operating table. I saw faces wearing surgical masks and moving quickly in silent choreography. The room was cold, the walls a light gray. It seemed everything was light, or reflections of light. My last thought before drifting into "anesthesia sleep" was, *The lights will help me find my way back.*

CHAPTER THIRTY-SEVEN

Real and Raw

My surgery lasted four long and intense hours.

Surgical oncologist Dr. Mark Landeros painstakingly worked to remove all of my breast tissue, along with the nipples. He carved out the inside of my chest, going deep near the chest wall, leaving the area concave. My breasts had shrunk, but he still managed to get close to two pounds from each side. He left a thin layer of loose skin, trying to remove every possible cancerous cell. Dr. Landeros also removed five lymph nodes that had lit up from the nuclear exam. Two lymph nodes from the right breast, and three from the left, were carefully removed, with all the tissue placed in steel containers. Those blobs of tissue and blood were sent to the lab to be examined, slice by slice, under a microscope.

Once the surgical team completed its work of removing the tissue, the next team moved in with different tools and a different goal. Plastic surgeon Dr. Frank Agullo arrived with several expanders to place on my exposed chest. He tried several sizes to find the best fit for my body. After choosing the perfect size, he filled them with blue saline solution and sewed up my new and much fuller breasts. Surgical tape covered the six-inch vertical scar on my lumpy chest. Off to the side, drains attached to small pumps skimmed off the excess fluid, and let it flow out of my body. My new breasts were squeezed into a surgical bra.

I opened my eyes in post-op to a beautiful sight: Carolina, sitting next to my bed, holding my hand. She had a reassuring smile, and her presence brought me peace. Jimmy was there, too, to plant three soft kisses on my forehead.

In and out of the groggy post-surgical sleep, I lifted my arms to check for mobility. I touched both breasts to make sure I still had some. As I reached to touch Stelhita, I began sobbing uncontrollably. I vividly felt my humanity in those precious moments, alive and loved, at my most vulnerable.

Jimmy knew that the waiting room was full of people who wanted to see me and make sure I was okay. He sprang into action and found a way to sneak them in. Making sure the nurse wasn't watching, he propped the door open and led them in, one by one, just to wave and let me know they were there; I wasn't alone. The nurse eventually caught him, and he got into trouble, but not before letting everyone in. Mission accomplished.

No amount of Propofol or other anesthesia drugs could ever erase the memories of that day—February 21st. How deeply painful it was for my family and friends to see me in a hospital bed, all so real and so raw.

The strong woman with the positive attitude shivered underneath the warm white hospital blankets. The white cotton gown sprinkled with blue designs, and opening to the back, was not enough to keep me warm. Knowing I had been sliced open, carved out, and sewn back together brought chills down my spine. As I gazed down the curve of my protruding new chest, my eyes were drawn to the end of the bed, and I saw the bright yellow socks on my feet. The hospital socks made me smile as I drifted back into a healing sleep.

I woke up with a clearer head to see Carolina, Marcos, Andres, and Arnoldo, my ex-husband, speaking softly with my dear friends Nicole and Griselda. Their conversations were indistinct, but I felt good knowing I had a room full of love.

Eventually, everyone but Carolina left. She and I remained sharing the four walls, along with hourly visits from the night nurses. With the oxygen cannula and the boots around my legs, we settled down for the night.

The rhythm of the post-surgery compression boots massaging my legs brought soothing relief as my breathing followed along. The pain medication helped numb my discomfort, and although my brain was fuzzy, there was still something very clear in my mind: My daughter's unconditional love and strength were all I needed to get me through that night. I recalled the first time I held her in my arms. She weighed 7 pounds 7 ounces and had a full head of hair. Carolina's love and compassion held me in her arms that night.

CHAPTER THIRTY-EIGHT

You Willed It Out of Your Soul

There is power in displaying a positive attitude when confronted with tragedy, pain, and suffering. But can you "will" out of your soul an illness such as bilateral breast cancer? Can the way you live life rid your body of cancer?

If you believe in miracles, the answer is, "Yes." Medical technology such as CT scans, MRIs, mammograms, and ultrasounds highlight and measure tumors. There are new and improved medications to fight breast cancer, and immunotherapy to help keep it at bay. But there's nothing to measure the soul.

The soul doesn't weigh anything, but I believe it is the literal life energy of your body. It's that feeling inside your chest and gut that guides your actions, behavior, and decisions.

Jimmy sent me these words via text message after doctors told me there was no longer cancer in my body: *You willed it out of your soul.*

This is a deeply profound phrase, just seven powerful words. It's hopeful, encouraging. Merriam-Webster (or Google, if you prefer) defines the soul as the moral and emotional nature of human beings. The definition seems simple to comprehend, but the soul really is so much more complex. Our souls are intangible, yet so alive if we allow them to soar.

What we experience as humans walking the earth can often feel soul-killing (e.g., death, disease, social ills). The list of things that can hurt your soul is long and painful.

Despite my career as a journalist, giving a voice to others, my voice was silenced when I was only ten years old. When I was in fourth grade, I was sexually assaulted, and my abuser said, "Don't tell anyone." My memory fails me, perhaps the pain blocked the assaults, but it took me many years to acknowledge what happened in my childhood. It wasn't until I was in my fifties that I spoke about it, and I finally began to heal. All those years, I felt dirty, shameful, guilty, and unworthy. My self-esteem shattered. My anger transformed into sadness and deep despair. I lived with that dirty little secret deep in my heart for decades.

I didn't like my body. I felt I was never thin enough and covered my arms and found ways to make my breasts look smaller by wearing loose dresses to hide the rolls around my waist and thick legs. I felt ugly. Later in life, I worked on my appearance to mask my broken spirit, feeling less of a girl, teenager, and woman.

Finally, at age 55, I felt safe enough and brave enough to reveal my secret during a woman's spiritual retreat. A weight and burden had been lifted off my shoulders. My soul began restoration.

Letting that secret out was liberating. I had forgiven my assailant, and I had forgiven myself. I told my children. I shared the news with my siblings and their wives and my closest friends. And now you know. I'm sharing this painful part of my life because I want you to know that we all have overcome challenges. I'm no different from you. Our souls cry out, and we must answer and nurture them.

When we lose a loved one, when a longtime relationship ends, or when we develop an illness, we are forever changed, altered. We feel broken to our core, deep into an area in our body and mind we can't fathom or seem to touch: our soul.

Sometimes, we bear the physical scars, reminding us of the impact, but there are other scars that aren't so visible or as quick to heal.

Our heart breaks into pieces, and we wonder if there's a way to piece it back together. The short and complicated answer is yes; many times we can piece together a heart, although it may never again be whole. It may keep breaking, to remind us not to close it up. But the soul, that's a different story. It can rebuild, renew. The soul possesses resilience, but with a catch. It must be tested for you to know it.

I had closed off a huge part of my life, and life, cancer, and suffering reminded me to open up again. What a test! What a challenge! In the middle of all the chaos and uncertainty, I can truthfully now say all the events in my life have been a blessing. I believe things happen for a reason. The reasons are still unfolding. God is showing me why.

And so, I must share my truth. I must share my brokenness. Did I will things out of my soul?

The answer is a resounding, "Yes!"

CHAPTER THIRTY-NINE

No Stripper Boobs!

Nine weeks after the double mastectomy, and after two fills with blue saline solution, it was time to drop the "gummy bear" implants into my breast pockets. That's the name I gave the cohesive silicone gel implants that would be the final surgical step on my breast cancer journey.

The six-inch vertical scars on my breasts had healed nicely. These implants were my best option, given that I only had a thin layer of skin left. I did a little bit of research on the kind of breasts I wanted, and I also came up with a name for those. Victoria's Secret breasts: perfect cleavage, round and perky. It's certainly not the best way to get a boob job, but I take my blessings where I find them.

It wasn't a particularly special day. The procedure was an exchange. Pockets of silicone material, which had made my skin expand enough for a size DD, would be popped open, drained of the blue saline liquid, and replaced with permanent implants.

I'd done my own investigation, as a curious and inquisitive reporter, into what the surgery actually looked like. It was sobering to see what the chest cavity looks like after a double mastectomy, before the expander or implant is placed in the pocket. It wasn't hard to see why some women would choose not to have reconstructive surgery. The process was daunting.

Plastic surgeon Dr. Frank Agullo reminded me, "This is the fun part of the painful process. You get to choose the size and shape of your new breasts."

⸻

Sandra and Marcos took me to the hospital that afternoon. I was Dr. Agullo's last surgery of the day. By now, I knew the drill behind the curtain by heart:

Strip down.

Change into the hospital gown.

Slip on the bright yellow socks.

Andres and his dad came to see me before the surgery. It was awkward, yet comforting, to see the two of them standing nervously at the edge of my bed. We were all nervous. There are so many risks involved in any kind of surgery (including death), a fact I was reminded of as I signed the consent forms. We all were wondering, for what seemed like the millionth time, about the risks of things going wrong in the OR.

Once again, certified registered nurse anesthetist, Lee Hunt, was there for us. Although there were fewer people in the room this time, she still led us in prayer, strengthening our resolve, leaning on our faith.

Covered in prayer, waiting to be taken to surgery, I took inventory of where I was at that moment. My hair had grown back to about a quarter inch long. I still wasn't quite ready for anyone to see what I looked like under Stelhita. I was quick to remind the medical team to not remove the wig, and to just tuck it into the surgical cap instead.

My eyelashes were also slowly coming back. Four months after the last chemo session, they were sprouting through the eyelids, little black dots poking through skin that had been barren. Oh, how I missed my long and curly lashes.

Having your femininity tested is tough. Is it vanity? The short answer is no. It hurts the psyche. Having your breasts cut off of your body . . . well, it's not supposed to happen, is it? Breasts don't define me, but they are part of who I am. My breasts had given sustenance to my three children. Now they were gone, and they were about to be replaced with implants made of highly cohesive gel.

There is so much to think about and absorb, beyond the idea of dying from cancer. It all seems so superficial, considering that cancer kills. All the time. But this, too, is a challenge and part of the process.

Dr. Agullo walked in sporting black scrubs with his logo embroidered on his chest, ready to work his magic.

I reminded him, "I don't want my breasts to be too big. I want them to be an appropriate size for my five-foot-two frame. And perky, I want perky round breasts with just enough cleavage to look sexy."

He stood next to me and listened.

I went on to say, "I don't want stripper boobs. I want 'Victoria's Secret model' boobs."

Dr. Agullo smiled all the way to his eyes, chuckled, and nodded. He already knew; oh, how he knew! I think I had told him dozens of times before in the office, "No stripper boobs!"

An hour later, I awoke in post-op. Marcos, Sandra, and Jimmy were at the foot of the bed. Not fully awake from the anesthesia, I sneaked a peek at my breasts. They were perfect. Dr. Agullo had made a bra with surgical tape, framing my beautiful breasts. Perfect. They didn't have nipples yet. Still perfect. There were no drains connected to my chest this time, and there was no need for me to stay overnight.

I was discharged at 10:00 p.m. As the sliding glass doors of the hospital opened for us to exit, I took in a deep breath of gratitude. I took another as Jimmy got me into Sandra's car, strapped on the seatbelt, and shared three kisses goodnight with me.

I was going home.

CHAPTER FORTY

New Nips!

They're darker than the rest of your skin. They're three dimensional. They become erect when cold or stimulated, and they pop out of your T-shirt if you're wearing the wrong bra!

Nipples aren't just for decoration or fun. They are the vessels that connect your milk to your hungry baby's stomach. When my kids were babies, I hooked up my breasts to an electric pump to suck out the milk and put it in a bottle. I nursed all three of my babies this way, pumping milk and freezing it in small plastic bags to heat up and feed them when I was at work.

Breasts are magical appendages! We may complain they're too big, too small, too round, or too soft, but when they're gone, you realize the importance they played in your life.

My breasts had been replaced, but my nipples had not. A few days before Christmas, I decided to gift myself some. Nipples aren't usually on a typical wish list, but they were at the top of mine. I was nervous, but also excited, about getting them tattooed.

———

I arrived early at the doctor's office and was whisked into a room.

The nurse handed me a white robe.

"I'll step out for a minute while you take off your bra. We need to take a few pictures," she said.

I quickly took off my bra and slipped on the robe.

"Ready?"

I said yes, then followed her into the room.

"Please take off your robe and stand straight, facing the camera. I need to get a full frontal," she said.

Click! Click! went the camera.

"Turn a quarter to your left."

Click.

"Now let's get a close up of your right breast," the nurse said.

Click. The left breast also got some close ups.

"We're done. You can follow me to the room," she added.

Once inside the room, I sat on the exam chair and bared my breasts. The nurse squeezed out some numbing cream and rubbed it on the area where the nipples would be drawn. I had always heard getting a tattoo was painful.

I thought to myself, *How much will it hurt?* After all the pain I've pushed through, I convinced myself that it would be a breeze! It couldn't possibly be more painful than the surgery that had carved out all the breast tissue in my chest! I was more than ready.

Ready to take one more step in the journey to try to feel and look normal.

My new normal.

I almost dozed off waiting for the tattoo artist to come in. It takes a while to numb the area. A knock on the door brought me right back to attention. It was the tattoo artist, Samantha, who walked in pushing a small metal cart. It held several small bottles of different shades of ink and a tattoo gun. Samantha wore latex gloves and scrubs, and she had several tattoos on her arms and chest area. She had a friendly smile, perfectly applied makeup, and thick fake eyelashes. I liked her at once.

"Hi, sorry to keep you waiting! Are you ready? I brought several shades of brown," she said.

"Hi," I answered, surprised to learn we would need several shades of brown.

I'd been advised to take pictures of my breasts before the double mastectomy to duplicate the size and color of the nipples and areolas.

I had done my homework, so I pulled up the picture on my phone and showed her.

"I can create something that will look similar by using different hues and shades," Samantha explained. "I will try my best to make them look natural and three dimensional."

"Let's do this!" I said with a nervous smile.

Samantha pulled out a marker and drew the circle. It wasn't a perfect circle because nipples aren't perfect! The imperfections show character and even personality! She drew in some areolas; then she measured the distance and height between the nipples to make sure they were high enough and in the middle of the breast.

"Do you like the color and size of the areola?" Samantha asked.

I considered the question, and thought, *Why not?*

"I would like them smaller, pre-children size," I answered.

With a knowing smile, Samantha erased the dotted circle with rubbing alcohol and redrew smaller, more dainty nipples.

Not too big. Not too small. Just right to highlight my perfectly round and perky breasts!

I picked a pecan brown. Not too dark. Not too light. Just right for my skin tone.

Samantha filled the gun with the ink, asked me to lie down on the big white leather chair, and began to work her magic.

She kept asking, "Are you okay? Do you need any more numbing cream?"

"I'm okay. I don't have any pain," I answered.

I could see the gun piercing the skin and depositing ink into my skin. It didn't hurt at first. And then it stung when the gun pierced deeper areas of the skin. Several areas of my breast seemed more sensitive than others.

I took deep breaths as she wiped down the area with a cotton ball.

It was a little bloody.

"At the tattoo parlor, we don't use numbing cream. We earn the tattoos with pain," Samantha said, her tattoo gun continuing its tiny punctures on my breasts.

She congratulated me, reminding me that I had earned mine way before that day, undergoing the double mastectomy. Yes, I'd put in enough pain to earn these new, perfect nipples.

"Let's check in the mirror so you can tell me what you think. We can go darker if you'd like?" Samantha asked.

"Let's go a tad darker," I answered, willing to endure the stinging sensation a little longer.

And then . . .

"All done. I'm going to put Saran Wrap and tape on your breasts to protect the skin from infection," Samantha told me as we finished up.

She reassured me they would be completely healed in two weeks, and she recommended I change out the plastic twice a day for four days.

"Don't soak your breasts when you shower and call me if you see any signs of infection. We can touch them up later," she said.

"Thank you," I answered as I attempted to put on my bra and blouse so I could head to work. After biopsies, chemo, immunotherapy, and surgery, my breasts had finally been returned to me.

CHAPTER FORTY-ONE

Dying with Dignity

After I was diagnosed with cancer, the path ahead was clear: fight.

The cancer in my breasts was removed. Chemo pushed other cancer cells into a dormant stage. The tumors in both breasts had been HER2 positive, meaning they contained a protein called human epidermal growth factor receptor. HER2 positive actually *promotes* the growth of cancer cells, and it's usually more aggressive than other types of breast cancer.

It's a hard reality I face every day, knowing that, in all likelihood, the cancer will come back, despite receiving the best cancer treatment available, the prayers, the good intentions, maintaining proper nutrition, having a positive attitude, and exercising and living a life of purpose. Cancer mutates; it's silent and stealthy until a PET scan finds its tentacles wrapped around your organs, including your brain. Often, breast cancer metastasizes to the lungs, liver, bones, and brain. I understand it can cause excruciating pain when it's in the bones and liver; it robs the oxygen from your lungs, and when it reaches your brain, it steals your essence, the very thing that makes you who you are.

When I was told I had cancer for a second time, I decided I wanted to live and fight. I didn't retreat. I faced it with fierce determination and faith. I gambled by waging a very public war, not knowing where the journey would lead me, and thousands followed. They prayed for me and cheered me on. I showed everyone that I wasn't going to let cancer define or beat me.

ESPN anchor Stuart Scott fought cancer of the appendix for seven years. He inspired my fight with these words, delivered in a powerful speech at the Espy Awards:

"When you die, that does not mean you lose to cancer. You beat cancer by how you live, why you live, and the manner in which you live."

Stuart died 6 months later at age 49. I don't know how he faced the last few days or who was with him or even if he was lucid. It doesn't matter. He won.

Cancer forces you to think about death, to think about *your* death. Cancer makes you dig deep into the essence of who you are, and not only how you want to live, but also how you want your journey to end. For me, winning that fight—living my life on my terms—also means dying on my own terms.

This is one of the hardest parts of the journey. It's not something I take lightly. I know that not everyone will agree with the conclusions I came to, and that's okay with me. I fought cancer with as much grace and dignity as I could, and with the help of my doctors. I will also die with grace and dignity, and with the help of a cocktail prescribed by a physician.

Whew! I have given it a voice and put it on paper.

Growing up Catholic, I was taught that suicide was considered a grave sin, that people who take their own lives don't get a proper Catholic burial and go straight to hell. No one wants to burn in hell! I don't want to burn in hell, but I also don't want to live in the hell cancer can cause. I don't want those who love me to live through the hell of seeing me waste away a day, hour, minute, or second at a time without control of my faculties.

I did my research.

I learned about Brittany Maynard, and her fight for assisted death after she was diagnosed with brain cancer at age 29. Brittany moved from California to Oregon to take advantage of Oregon's Death with Dignity law. Brittany ended her life with drugs prescribed by a doctor in October 2014, 10 months after her diagnosis. In 2014, California was not a state where physician-assisted suicide was legal. California has now joined 9 other states that allow medical aid in dying, and they are Colorado, the District of Columbia, Hawaii, Montana, Maine, New Jersey, Oregon, Vermont, and Washington. Lawmakers in New Mexico, which is a few miles away from my home, have been debating whether to make physician-assisted death legal for several years. Texas does not have a Death with Dignity law.

Life, and now cancer, have helped me search and find a part of myself and the courage I never knew I had. That courage includes the decision to move to a state that allows terminally ill patients to die with dignity. If the cancer in my body returns, and won't back down, like it did this time, I will pack my bags and go to a place with breathtaking sunsets, taking in my last breath, surrounded by love and memories. Just like Stuart Scott, I will win in life . . . and in death.

CHAPTER FORTY-TWO

Stell's Bold Journey

He stands six feet tall and has a pink nose, two white socks on his back legs, and a pleasant disposition. His coat is brown and shiny, and his tail and mane are the shade of dark chocolate. He's soft to the touch. He tips the scales at one thousand pounds of muscle and might.

Stell's Bold Journey is a Bay Thoroughbred. He's the son of Atilla's Storm, New Mexico's top sire for 2017 and 2018. His mother is Bold Jubilation, also a stakes-winning mare. As with all thoroughbreds, Stell's Bold Journey carries part of his momma's name. Tradition. Blood. Promise. Just like his full brother, Stormin' the Jewels, Stell's Bold Journey promises to be a stakes-winning racehorse. He's won more than a half a million dollars already.

He's also my namesake.

Bold.

Courageous.

That's how Jimmy describes my public and private journey with bilateral breast cancer.

Graceful.

Determined, like a racehorse that pushes through, passing the other horses on the track to make his way to the front. The leader. No photo finish, just the clear winner, earning the coveted spot at the winner's circle, and wearing a blanket of 554 red roses from the Kentucky Derby. Stell's Bold Journey could be posing for pictures and smiling after a 2-kilometer race.

I didn't quite understand the significance of this gift until I saw and touched Stell's Bold Journey. We first met when he was a weanling, in one of the stalls on Jimmy's farm. I didn't know what to expect because I'm not particularly comfortable around animals because I didn't grow up around them. I don't remember having a pet dog. We had canaries and mocking birds when I was growing up, but you can't pet or train them!

He was with his momma, Bold Jubilation, who was protecting him and nursing him into a yearling. Stell's Bold Journey had long, wobbly legs. He would peek his head out, cautious, but curious, behind his mom. Stell's Bold Journey was born with a purpose, but he needed time to grow into it.

We were reacquainted three days before he was loaded on a trailer, headed to Ruidoso Downs for auction. It was a beautiful summer morning in El Paso as we headed out to A&A Ranch in Anthony, New Mexico. It's next to the river levee. The water flowed calmly, and the brush along the banks was green and lush. There wasn't a cloud in the beautiful blue sky. It seemed a perfect day to give my send-off to the horse I'd watched turn from a baby to a teen.

Stell's Bold Journey's groomer saw me and Jimmy drive up in a big truck. He brought the now stately horse over to say hello. I noticed his graceful stride and calm disposition. He has a swagger about him. Perhaps he knows who his mom and dad are, so he walks proudly!

On his left side, he sported a gold name plate on his leather halter, engraved with "Stell's Bold Journey" in bold black letters. A tag with his hip number—67—was visible on the right side. He looked at me with his big brown eyes and leaned his nose toward me to embrace me and identify my scent.

He said hello! Buenos días. He's bilingual. His handlers speak to him in English and Spanish. He made me smile, and I felt relaxed and comfortable touching him. I rubbed his cheek and petted his strong jawline. His neck was thick and strong. His brown hair gleamed, shiny and healthy. His groomer told us that Stell's Bold Journey has a proportioned body with defined thigh muscles and a powerful loin and backside.

His trainer Juan said, "He has a powerful motor and transmission. But most importantly, he has a good disposition to learn and follow commands. En Ingles y Español. Es muy inteligente."

Juan gave me the reins, and we walked toward the round pen. Stell's Bold Journey was warmed up and ready to run. Juan loosened his halter, and he began to trot gracefully and then run. His massive body stretched and moved in cadence. He was majestic! He ran and kicked up dirt, leaving a cloud of dust in his path. His mane flapped in the wind, and his galloping was so perfect that it seemed choreographed. Stell's Bold Journey glistened in the sunlight as he ran past me. He was showing off, but he knew his mission: To run for a cause. To run with purpose.

Jimmy had brought him to this stable to get proper nutrition and exercise to become a racehorse. He was well on his way. We got a tour of the rest of the ranch and barns. On our way out, I stopped to say goodbye, good luck, and thank you!

I whispered in his ear, "Okay, little boy, you're going to do well at the auction." I gave Stell's Bold Journey a kiss, and he leaned over and gave me a kiss on my arm.

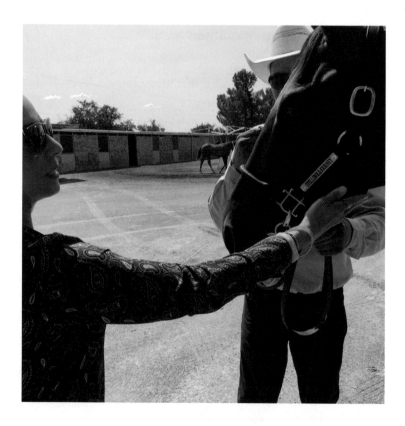

I would see him a few days later. He, along with hundreds of other thoroughbreds and quarter horses, were auctioned off at the Ruidoso Yearling sale at Ruidoso Downs Racetrack and Casino.

The day was sunny, but as we neared Ruidoso, it began to rain. It was wet, gray, and foggy. Despite the gloomy outdoors, the big barn was filled with excitement. There were bays, browns, grays, sorrels, and blacks. We spotted Stell's Bold Journey in his stall. His name and description were on a piece of paper taped on the outside of his stall. His trainer had attached a pink ribbon on the paper with his name. He came over to say hello. I could tell he recognized my scent. I hope he recognized my heart.

Stell's Bold Journey was ready. He had been lovingly cared for, and protected, by his mother, the grooms at Jimmy's JD IV Farms in Canutillo, and by the trainers at A&A Ranch. He was born to race, and to win. It's in his blood. Did he know why he was in Ruidoso? I believe he did.

It was time to go to the auction.

The sun was setting, and the crowd was getting excited as Jimmy and I walked around the barn, sizing up the other yearlings. We flipped through the pages of the catalogue, learning about other horses' lineages. Jimmy was nervously excited. His investments of time and money on this horse were about to come to fruition.

Who would give Stell's Bold Journey a chance to develop, to groom him into a stakes winner? Who else would believe in his heart? I watched Stell's Bold Journey strut into the auction barn. He was showing off as he pranced in the dirt, flaunting his ancestry. Stell's Bold Journey was showing the spectators his potential and drive to win.

I was nervous. As the auctioneer introduced him, I began recording on my cell phone. I felt everything around me had stopped moving. My eyes were zeroed in on Stell's Bold Journey. The opening bid was $1,500. I lost sight of Stell's Bold Journey as he was led into the auction area, but I kept track of the numbers on the board. They kept changing. The person in charge of updating the numbers on the board couldn't keep up. The auctioneer's voice was hypnotizing. It was monotone, but with a rhythm that wouldn't stop until the bidders nodded their heads, agreeing to pay more money.

I blinked back tears, which then rolled down my cheeks. I held the camera steady to capture the sights and sounds. It was happening so fast. The number kept going up. I kept crying. My eyelashes were already ungluing, but I didn't care if they fell off. The bidding stopped, and the final amount popped up on the board: $40,000! My quiet cry turned into a subdued sob. Just two minutes of bidding, and Stell's Bold Journey was auctioned for forty grand to someday benefit the Stand with Estela fund. A rush of different emotions filled my head and heart. I felt relief, surprise, happiness, and awe!

Stell's Bold Journey commanded a high price, but to me, he'll always be priceless. I can't put a price tag on his message of hope and determination, on the inspiration he gave me, as I made my own journey through breast cancer to survival. The value of that is more precious than any amount of money to me.

Stell's Bold Journey lives in Fort Hancock now, about a four-hour drive from El Paso, poised to make his mark on the world.

CHAPTER FORTY-THREE

Circle of Love

Why did I write this book? I ask myself that question every time I put my hands and fingers on the keyboard. Every time I read what I've written, I ask myself, *What's the point of sharing my story?*

Like everything in this journey, the reasons why have slowly revealed themselves. I don't consider myself special or extraordinary. I am passionate about doing what I believe in my heart is right. I am passionate about doing anything I can do to help my family and friends heal from what they've seen me go through. I am passionate about helping my community, my cancer sisters and their families, stricken with this devastatingly challenging disease, to heal and find the courage to push through each day. My journey encouraged me to open up and share my story of finding, accepting, and sharing love and all its nuances.

This is a love story.

It's a love story between me, my three children, two siblings, and close relatives. It's a love story between friends who have lifted me through this journey. It's a love story of two broken souls, brought together by God, to emerge whole again. It's a love story about coworkers who saw the worst—and best—of me, and still loved what they saw. It's a love story of strangers—my beloved community—coming together in support of a woman they've allowed in their homes via their televisions almost every day for thirty-seven years.

As a journalist, I've learned that my job as a storyteller is also to educate, so here's the first lesson on love. I looked this up so I could better understand what I experienced, and continue to experience, during this life lesson, and I want to share it with you.

The Greeks knew what they were talking about! Now that I fully understand, I am embracing and living all the types of love they defined.

AGAPE LOVE

It's selfless, a love bigger than ourselves. It's a love that accepts, forgives, trusts, and believes. It is defined as "the highest form of love, charity" and "the love of God for (wo)man, and the love of (wo)man for God."

I define it as a love which guides my spirituality and the acknowledgment of God in my life. I've always been a spiritual person, but this part of my being flourished as I was confronted with a life-threatening disease. I extended my hand to God. He grabbed it and patiently and lovingly walked me through this journey. He never let go, and He actually gave me many other hands to hold along the way. He placed everyone in my path for a reason. I trusted my physicians because I knew He was guiding them. I knew my children would be okay because He was in charge of making sure they were being taken care of. I turned all my fears and hope to Him. I am forever grateful for my circle of love, which starts with God in the center.

STORGE LOVE

This is the love my three children and I share, an intangible, unbreakable bond that can be communicated just as much with a stern look as it can with a kind glance, a loving smile, or a warm embrace. It's unconditional love that is nurturing and sublime. For me, it's the truest love on Earth, shared between a mother and the children she carried in her womb and essence. Carolina, Marcos, and Andres are the reason my heart is full of gratitude.

PHILIA

The love that's shared between friends. I have a handful of friends. Some go back decades, while others don't even go back five years. No matter the time, they're all deep and meaningful relationships. We've shared the loss of parents, failed marriages, lost pregnancies, and many successes. I care deeply for these women, whom I consider the sisters I never had.

PRAGMA

Enduring love is a partnership described as an effort from both sides to offer each other patience, tolerance, acceptance, honor, and respect. I share that with everyone in my life. I have learned to not be so judgmental because I, too, have made many mistakes along the way.

PHILAUTIA

Philautia is self-love, a love I describe as feeling comfortable in your own skin. It's the ability to love oneself fully, knowing one must, in order to love others well. When a person lacks self-love, this can lead to MANIA (obsessive love) that seeks *external* validation of the self, rather than *internal* acceptance of the self, through healthy self-esteem. It's taken me decades, but I continue to carve a place in my heart for me.

EROS

Oh! The sweet love between two people who come together and feel fiery passion for one another, whole, worthy, and deserving.

Love is a verb that I want to live every day. I refuse to allow the tragedy of an illness to rob me of my ability to love fully. Love, and all the magical moments I've lived with the people I love and who love me, is all I will take with me when I die.

I choose to live purposefully, with love.

I choose to love intentionally and truly.

I choose to laugh harder, with love.

Every. Single. Day.

CHAPTER FORTY-FOUR

Not Everyone Has a Happy Ending

Not everyone has a happily ever after. For now, I am cancer-free and hope to stay that way until I'm not.

Fighting cancer requires a mentally, physically, and medically aggressive plan and team of family, friends, and physicians. Here are some tips.

When you find a lump in your breast, don't panic. Call and make an appointment to see your doctor. He or she will examine you and order a mammogram or ultrasound. You may need a needle biopsy which will help confirm a diagnosis.

If you are diagnosed with breast cancer find out the type: Estrogen + or -, Progesterone + or - and HER2 + or -.

The type of cancer will determine the course of treatment.

You'll need to get an MRI and possibly a PET scan to determine if the cancer has spread.

Ask about the course of treatment and the medications you'll be administered. Not all cancers are treated with chemotherapy or radiation. If your doctor prescribes chemotherapy ask about Neulasta to help reduce the risk of infection, which is administered in a patch on your hip or arm and delivers the drug 24 hours after each treatment.

Ask if you'll need surgery: mastectomy or lumpectomy.

If you will need a mastectomy, you'll have to consider having reconstructive surgery; you'll have to choose between implants or DIEP flap surgery that uses your own tissue from either your back, thighs, or stomach area. If you don't undergo reconstruction surgery, you can obtain a silicone or non-silicone prosthesis you can wear under a special bra. There are specialty shops.

Nipples. If you have them removed you'll need to find a tattoo artist who creates three-dimensional nipples.

Don't believe everything you read on the internet. Let it be a resource and only visit credible websites. The most reliable resources are your local hospitals and regional cancer centers. The National Cancer Institute has pertinent and updated information. Websites that end in .edu or .gov are more reliable.

Don't believe you'll have the same journey or outcome as your friend or relative. Everybody is different and battles cancer differently.

Journaling is critical. Writing down how you are feeling is liberating and cathartic. Your memory will likely fail you, so write down everything and keep it as a physical file or a dedicated file on your computer. List all the medications you're taking.

Go shopping for a wig before you need it. It will need to be cut and styled by a professional. There are synthetic hair wigs and wigs made from human hair. Buy a couple. Synthetic hair is easy to manage because it doesn't lose its shape and is wash-and-wear.

Wigs made from human hair require more care and are more expensive. Wigs start at $50 and can run into the thousands.

If you require chemotherapy and radiation your skin will get dry. You'll need to moisturize with a noncomedogenic cream or lotion.

Your mouth will produce less saliva. Use a special mouthwash.

Carry a change of clothes in case you have an emergency.

Chemotherapy can cause severe diarrhea.

Stay active with brisk walking and using light weights. You may lose weight along with muscle.

Learn to listen to your body. Allow yourself to be vulnerable and accept all the help that is offered to you.

Your medical team will be an oncologist, surgical oncologist, and plastic surgeon. Develop a relationship with all medical personnel, especially your oncology nurses. They see cancer every day.

Pray and strengthen your personal relationship with God, family, and friends. They will be your lifelines.

Open up your heart, have a positive attitude, and find beauty and magic in everything you see and do.

Dusty Rose: The Road to the Future

She stands 52 inches tall, with a carbon frame and hydraulic disc brakes.

When I saw her for the first time—a 2021 Specialized Tarmac SL7 Expert Ultegra Di2—she was hanging from the ceiling at Crazy Cat Cyclery on Stanton Street in West El Paso. The shop owner, Roberto Barrio, carefully lifted her off the hooks and gently set her down right next to me.

She took my breath away.

Her name is Dusty Rose. She's a performance bicycle, and she's absolutely beautiful. She's also intimidating as hell.

Jimmy ordered this bike months ago, and today, she finally arrived. He helped pick out the best medium-sized pedals, a bottle cage, tracker, and a bag for tools just in case I get a flat tire. There's even just enough room to slip in hot pink lipstick! We walked around the store picking out accessories.

"Do you want the geometry grail glove or the long finger gloves?" Jimmy asked. "You need padding, so the full finger gloves are probably better," he added.

I nodded, politely agreeing.

"Do they come in pink?" I asked.

"Do you have shorts with padding that look like you're wearing a diaper?" Jimmy asked.

"I have a few," I answered.

"Pick whatever you want. I don't recommend we get you pedals with clips or clip-on shoes. You have to graduate to those."

I thought to myself, *The road to graduation is a long one, and I haven't even gotten back on the saddle.* Bicycle seats are called saddles, just like the ones on a horse.

My eyes skimmed her beautiful pink frame, and I smiled inside.

The bike technician lifted Dusty Rose away and placed her on a special platform to get her ready for me to ride.

Jimmy made friendly talk with the tech as I walked nervously throughout the store, trying to figure out how I was going to do that. Anxiety built in my mind as I tried to remember how I found myself in this place.

Jimmy had ordered a bike for me, and one for himself, as Christmas gifts. Mine came in early, but his bike was on backorder for a couple of months. Jimmy started cycling when I was diagnosed, and he has since become an avid indoor and outdoor cyclist.

"Your bike is ready, Ms. Casas; let's try it out," Robert said excitedly.

Under my breath, I said, "Oh shit, how am I going to pull this off?"

Jimmy followed as I walked outside, attempting to camouflage my nerves.

He said proudly, "I got you this because you are a two-time cancer survivor. It's perfect for you."

I smiled, but inside I was so afraid of disappointing him and myself.

I could feel my heart pounding out of my chest, and my head started spinning. My palms were sweaty, and my eyes started watering. I was in doubt of my ability to ride Dusty Rose!

Robert was already on his bike, balancing Dusty Rose, waiting for me to get on and get going. It was just going to be us, taking a short ride, so I could get a feel for her, and try out the brakes and gears. We were in the bike lane on busy Stanton Street, facing a fork in the road ahead. The symbolism wasn't lost on me. *You have a choice to make, Estela*, I thought to myself.

Out of the corner of my eye, I caught Jimmy observing the moment. He looked so handsome in his white shirt, blue jeans, and cowboy boots! I reluctantly looked away to focus on the challenge ahead. Swinging my left leg over the frame, I climbed on. She felt right. Dusty Rose was not too tall, and not too short; she was just right for my short legs and five-foot-one frame.

"Okay, Estela, let's do this. We'll go straight past Albertsons, and then we'll turn right onto the street up ahead," said Robert as he took off slowly ahead of me.

I froze. I couldn't move. It was as if my legs were strapped to the concrete underneath.

"I can't do this," I told Robert.

Robert cycled back around and got off his bike. He straddled Dusty Rose's front tire, leaned into me, and said, "You can do this. Relax and just push off and start pedaling. You're going to love the ride."

I looked straight back at him, feeling tears swell in my eyes, hidden behind my sunglasses. I sobbed quietly, wanting to make sure Jimmy didn't see me break down. I squeezed my hands tightly on the handlebars, and in between the tears I responded, "I don't deserve this bike."

Robert's eyebrows went up, surprised at what he was hearing.

"Why would you say that?" he asked. "Of course, you deserve this bike! Jimmy wants you to ride the best, and he picked this pink bike especially for you."

I felt like I was ten years old all over again, a ten-year-old child who didn't want to fall or fail. I'd fallen so badly, a few years ago while biking in Oregon, that I broke two ribs. At that time, I felt like I wasn't good enough for this magnificent bike, because I hadn't really been on a bike since the accident. I wasn't sure I could handle it.

"I don't want to disappoint him," I said.

Robert leaned in closer and said, "You won't disappoint him. I know exactly how you feel. I've owned this shop for years, and I've been riding for years, and my companion is a better cyclist. I've learned to accept that. You're going to be just fine, and you can share another thing in common with Jimmy. He's an excellent cyclist, but you don't have to compete with him, compete with yourself."

I wiped my tears. His words of validation gave me wings, and the courage, to not let the fear of failure prevent me from living. I had allowed doubt and fear to paralyze me so many times! I had been through too much already to allow a bicycle to control my emotions.

And then, by the grace of God and a puff of wind, I was able to place my right foot on the pedal. Left, right. Left, right. Soon, I was pedaling my way up Stanton street, putting my fear into action, and making it work for me. Another challenge met.

Robert got ahead of me, and he kept looking back to make sure I was okay.

"How does the bike feel?" he called back to me.

"Amazing!" I called back. "I feel like I'm riding on a cloud. It's liberating and empowering!"

Sunlight warmed my face, and the slight breeze messed up my short hair. I was flying again. When I am facing a challenge and can't make a decision, I feel like I'm at the edge of a cliff, my feet teetering yet afraid to take that step and jump. I took the plunge, grew wings, and began flying again.

Jimmy's goal may have been to get me to ride again with "Las Picosas," and eventually to ride with him, but his gift represents so much more. Dusty Rose is helping me get back into something I enjoyed pre-cancer. As I was riding, I felt the picosa begin stirring again in my heart.

She will help me reclaim the things I unknowingly set aside when cancer came for me again. She and I will accomplish that, one ride at a time, as we ride forward into the future. Dusty Rose and I took the right path at that fork in the road. We both knew it could get bumpy later on down the road, with perhaps greater obstacles than heavy traffic and bad weather. Dusty Rose is ready to weather the storms in my journey, and so am I.

TEAM ESTELA: CAROLINA
GARLIC SHRIMP AND BUTTERED BISCUITS

August 2017.

I had just started a new job, traveling Monday through Thursday, living in a hotel, and trying to make sense of my mom's recent diagnosis. Being in the medical field, I believed it was necessary to get a second opinion. I encouraged my mom to seek advice at MD Anderson Cancer Center, and she agreed.

I drove four hours to Houston and picked her up at the airport. I had seen her two weeks before, when she'd received the Gold Nugget award from UTEP. As I spotted her from a distance at the airport, I noticed she was thinner. Despite that, Mom was wearing a wig, big earrings, and heels in typical Stel style, remaining focused and positive.

MD Anderson is a well-oiled machine. Although Texas Oncology and Dr. Valilis had transferred all her records, MD Anderson still needed to start their own medical file. So, Mom was whisked away to measure her arms in case she got edema from chemo and surgery. She had a new mammogram, and then an ultrasound, as I waited nervously in the family waiting room.

It took all day, but we were happy to hear the good news that Mom was receiving the best care possible in El Paso. The doctors at MD Anderson agreed with the protocols, and we walked out knowing we were doing everything in our power to fight to obtain good results.

It had been a long day for both of us, emotionally and physically exhausting, but it wasn't over yet. Mom wanted to buy a better-quality wig to wear on air, so I Googled the location of the wig shop she had chosen, and we hurried over. We got there just a few minutes before it was scheduled to close. We told Mom's story to the saleslady, and she got right to work, finding the perfect wig, shampoo, and conditioner for her. We walked out feeling blessed and accomplished.

The day was long, and we hadn't eaten. I was craving seafood, although Mom didn't have much of an appetite. Even though we'd had a lot of success that day, we needed time to breathe, catch up, and replenish ourselves.

We ordered food, and Mom ordered her usual: "I'll have a glass of Malbec," she said. I ordered my usual, too, a beer. All the activity of the day, all the tests, all the boxes that had to be checked, came flooding back to us after just a few sips of our drinks. In the middle of all the small talk, we both broke down and came to each other with honesty. Mom was feeling guilty about developing cancer. She said: "I'm sorry I have become a burden," as tears rolled down her sunken-in cheeks. She had lost so much weight. I was feeling overwhelmed by the uncertainty and fear of losing my mom to cancer. Mom wasn't a burden, and even in her darkest and most vulnerable moments she's strong and independent.

I cried and couldn't speak, but expressing all of those feelings was exactly what we needed to do. That evening, in a strange city, we left all our tears, fears, and doubts on the table with the garlic shrimp and buttered biscuits. From that day forward, we both knew we would fight like hell.

TEAM ESTELA: MARCOS
SHE MAKES IT LOOK EASY

My mom is tough. She's so tough, she makes tough things look easy.

But when I found out she was going to have to battle cancer a second time, I worried that it might break her. She—and we—had been through so much already. My parents' divorce had taken a toll on us all. Even though she's "mom" to me, to everyone else out there, she was Estela Casas. She loved her work, bringing the news to the El Paso/Las Cruces community, and she was damn good at it. My concern was that the demands of her job would make it harder for her to fight cancer again.

I had just graduated from Truman State University in Kirksville, Missouri, where I'd attended on a football scholarship. I had already decided to take a year off to figure out what I wanted to do, and I was studying for the GRE to get into a Physical Therapy program. I was working at a PT clinic with Sandra, my mom's close friend, and I felt I was finding my place in the world. But Mom's diagnosis left me feeling that the world was turned upside down.

My mom met me outside the house as I was getting home

after work. She told me, "I have cancer in both breasts," and said that my sister, Carolina, would be coming to town the following day.

I stared at her and remained silent. In fact, I didn't say much throughout this journey. I prefer to show my support, rather than say it, if you know what I mean.

Mom's always been strong, always guided us with discipline and held us to high standards. I know she does everything with love, tough love, but I wasn't prepared to see her apply that same tough love to herself.

I never questioned her decision to share her story on television, but sometimes it shocked me how open she was about her—and our—journey. It wasn't that our privacy was at risk. She always protected us—always. It was how she allowed herself to be vulnerable to judgments, to other people's opinions, and *not* for herself! She felt that if she could make a difference for others facing a diagnosis like hers, then she was doing her best, being her best.

I am proud she started the Stand with Estela fund because I think it shows how her choice to be so vulnerable is actually a strength. It has blessed us in numerous ways. So many people were looking out for her and worried about her health, and worried about how I would do through the process. "How's your mom doing?" friends would call and ask me. They would ask me how I was doing too. Her strength helped us through the tough times.

We shared so many special moments during her chemo, including the day Mom and Sandra were honored as UTEP Gold Nuggets. My uncle and godfather, Fernando, stood with me as we watched Mom walk toward the stage and receive her award. UTEP

President Dr. Diana Natalicio hugged my mom and thanked her for her service to UTEP and the community. I was so proud of her.

But maybe the most important moment for me was the day I took her to her third chemotherapy treatment. When she settled in her recliner and the nurse inserted the needle in her port-a-cath, she presented me with a long list of errands for me to run, including getting the oil changed in her car and buying groceries for the house. I had thought I was going to have to stay and keep her company, but I was wrong.

Mom didn't let a single treatment stop her from running the household and making sure my brother and I had food at the house. When I came back with a trunk full of groceries and clean oil running through the car motor, Mom was talking and laughing with the people next to her, who were also hooked up to an IV.

That's my mom. She makes everything look easy.

TEAM ESTELA: ANDRES
TRANSFORMATION

I've always wondered what growth and transition meant. I had seen my friends and family go through different challenges in their lives but never thought I would go through one myself. It was 2017 and the summer before eighth grade that would change my life forever. My mom had been diagnosed with breast cancer. I quickly became the kid who no longer watched everyone's lives change. I became one of them. I asked myself some difficult questions. Am I ready to see my mom go through this? Is this cancer fatal? Am I going to grow up without a mom? I was only 13 at the time and didn't have answers and really didn't know what a cancer diagnosis meant. My family and I are members of the Catholic Church. I had a relationship with God but not one where I would listen to His word and feel enlightened after a Sunday sermon. We had gone to church as a family after the news but the mood seemed different. I really can't explain it but everything seemed positive. I felt as if the church seemed brighter. This was a bit confusing after learning my mom was sick. I remember one Sunday looking up to my family members and each one had the same expression on their faces: the unexplainable look of hope. Fast forward to December 28th, 2017. It was Mom's last chemotherapy treatment and patients celebrate by ringing a bell at the cancer center. Mom rang the bell three times and each time I felt it was a testament that my mom is a fighter and always will be. I knew in that very moment that she was going be around to celebrate my life events and remind me to live each day with a greater purpose. I had now come closer to the definition of growth and transition. I grew as a person and was transitioning into a different phase in my life. I learned from watching her and my family that life is too short to sit around and let the world go by. I developed a love of volleyball during Mom's journey. I am living in Dallas, Texas, playing volleyball for an elite club team at 17. The best part about this sport is not only the great memories, but also knowing that my mom is around to see me spike the ball. I am so grateful to have her as a mentor, cheerleader, and simply Mom.

TEAM ESTELA: FERNANDO
CORAZÓN ROTO

On August 26, 2017, I happened to be in El Paso to play at an annual four-day golf tournament with my high school buddies. I spent a day with Estela and my two nephews before heading out to Ruidoso, New Mexico, for Curada Cincha. Curada Cincha is a golf outing for boys who were in the 1960s El Paso Boys Club. This was the 27th annual.

Upon my return, I noticed that Estela's usually upbeat demeanor had changed. It didn't take long for her to tell me of her cancer diagnosis. I was devastated.

I was angry, confused, and desperate, but mostly scared. My anger was directed at the situation. Why her, why now? She had only recently begun to get her life back after a long overdue divorce. She was only now starting to enjoy new experiences that made her happy.

Was this some kind of a test, for her, for the family? Whatever it was I was convinced that she did not deserve it. My confusion was due largely to how to proceed. I knew about the many deaths due to breast cancer but I did not know of the options or treatments available and I could not become an expert in the time that we were forced to make life-changing decisions. Like many men, I am a problem solver. I felt desperation because I wanted to fix everything, but quickly learned that I alone could not do it. I was scared because I only focused on the worst-case outcomes. I could see our lives changing for the worse and instead of focusing on the possible positives. I was paralyzed with fear. Yet, as the older brother, I could not show any of my feelings. I had to be a reliable shoulder for her to cry on and to provide insightful, wise, and workable solutions like other times in the past.

Estela has always had my unflinching support in any situation but this time I felt that my support was crucial. My niece Carolina had flown into town immediately and now the three of us would rush through the seven stages of grief in a period of days. We had no time to waste if we were to fight this monster. Amazingly, a workable short-term plan emerged. Mostly, it was knowledge that Estela had gathered over the years of support of women's health, Carolina's understanding of the medical system and how it works, and several outstanding doctors that set the course of treatment. I acted more like a cheerleader and a sounding board but my input was appreciated. The tests were scheduled, the doctor's appointments were made, and a treatment plan had started. What followed is a battle that rages on even now. My feelings of inadequacy and helplessness were assuaged. I flew home a few days later.

Estela's treatments had already begun when I returned to El Paso to accompany her at an event where she was named a UTEP Gold Nugget. I will never forget just how glamorous she looked that weekend wearing her new wig. But it was what happened at her home before the gala that will live in my heart and in my soul forever.

I had noticed she had started losing her hair after her first chemotherapy treatment. That day, she asked me to cut what was left. "I can't fix my hair. Can you just cut it off? There's not much left," she said.

My corazón broke. "Sure," I answered with hesitation, as she handed me the scissors. We got in front of the bathroom mirror and I started clipping. The silence was deafening as I carefully clipped away a few strands. But I had to stop. "No puedo," I said. I couldn't stomach seeing her completely bald.

"No worries," Estela said with a smile and parts of her scalp exposed, as she walked to her bedroom to pull her wig out of the box. I watched as she attached some double-sided tape on her forehead and carefully adjusted her wig. She said with a half-grin: "No one but me and you know how it really looks underneath." I also flashed a half-grin.

If it hadn't been for her acceptance, commitment, and complete trust in her treatment, I would have broken down in the small bathroom. It was only later that night after a beautiful dinner with friends and after a couple of martinis, that my efforts to maintain a strong demeanor collapsed. Looking back at the moment, I was embarrassed, but who was there to comfort me? Estela.

The pain, desperation, and the foreboding became part of Estela's life. But she did something that still stuns me when I think about it. She decided to share those feelings, those highly personal experiences not only with other women diagnosed with cancer but also with a wider audience of her many thousands of nightly news watchers. She established the STAND WITH ESTELA CASAS CANCER FOUNDATION to educate women about breast cancer and raise money to disburse to women who would otherwise not be able to afford aspects of their cancer treatment. Estela ordered thousands of bracelets engraved with her logo.

I too believe in her mission to educate so I contribute to the foundation and have worn the STAND WITH ESTELA pink bracelet from day one. It's now faded but it's a testament to Estela's promise to soldier on. 'P'alante!

I wear it proudly and it's a conversation starter with those who notice it on my wrist. It's an opportunity for me to raise awareness and share our journey, nuestra jornada, with breast cancer.

The pink rubber bracelet is also a constant reminder of one of the worst periods in my life. Those first few months after Estela's diagnosis were life-changing for me.

I now find it easier to be vulnerable. I have learned that strength and support can be given just by listening. It also reaffirmed my belief that you should never give up in your struggles to survive. The bracelet also reminds me of how the situation made my relationship with my sister so much stronger. This new bond is not only based on sibling love but also on mutual respect, trust, and knowledge that we are unconditionally there for each other. Hermanos!

TEAM ESTELA: TROY BELCHER
BALD IS BEAUTIFUL

On the first day of first grade, I was lucky enough to meet my best friend, Marcos Hernandez. From that day forward, we were almost always together, he at my house, or me at his. To this day, we do everything together, from riding quads to skiing to just hanging out. We're lucky to have been friends for most of our lives.

Our friendship naturally meant our families became close, too, so I've spent lots of time with Marcos's mother, Estela Casas.

Estela would take us to school in the morning; she cooked us great food and laughed at our jokes—no matter how ridiculous we probably sounded sometimes. We have so many memories together; it's hard to remember them all. However, I am going to share one of the best memories I have of the three of us.

At the end of the summer in 2017, Marcos broke the tough news about his mother's illness to me. I felt so proud of his strength and his actions during this moment because he was handling the situation with faith and positivity. I was finishing my last semester of college in Tucson, Arizona at the time, so it hurt me that I could not be there to support their family. I began to think about what I could do to bring some relief to them, to let them know I had their backs. I knew chemo was definitely in Estela's future, so the idea of shaving my head kept popping into my mind. The decision was tough. I had never realized how much I valued my hair, but I shared a moment with Estela that would change my mind and heart forever.

That fall, I came home to visit my family, and I stopped by to check on Marcos. For weeks, I had been joking about letting Estela shave my head. The night before shaving my head, we were eating in Estela's kitchen when I asked her to remove her scarf. After a little hesitation, she agreed. My heart broke to see the sadness that overtook her face. She seemed embarrassed, because she did not have her signature hair sitting on top of her head. In that moment, all the fear I had about losing my own hair was gone, and I knew I wanted to do this for her.

The next day, we all gathered in the same kitchen, plugged in the clippers, and were off. The moment felt great. We were laughing and making jokes, and at times, becoming emotional. Estela did most of the work, and Marcos took lots of photos. The simplicity of the shaving helped the three of us psychologically in ways we did not see coming. It was important to me for Estela to feel beautiful, even during that difficult time.

Over the next several weeks, I was continuously asked why I had shaved my head. Every time I told the story to a friend, a teacher, or even a stranger, I felt fulfilled that something so small could have such an impact. I only hoped that the simple act could spread awareness and influence more people to support the women of October.

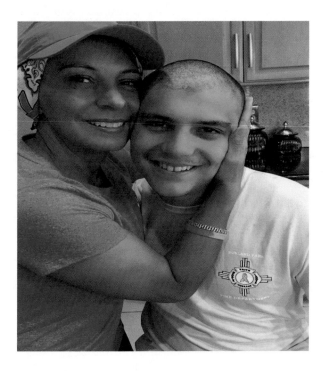

TEAM ESTELA: SANDRA
THINGS HAPPEN FOR A REASON

From the moment I met Estela, we shared an immediate sisterly bond. Stell was in a great spiritual, emotional, and physical state of mind. (I'm one of only a handful who calls her Stell!) The trip to Washington, DC was transformative for her. After the initial examination in the hotel room where I found a lymphatic cord, with 4 enlarged lymph nodes in her armpit and arm, I didn't have the courage to examine her breast because finding the tumors would have ruined the remaining three days of the trip.

Stell was unshaken and pressed forward despite our cancer conversation and actually went into *Estela KVIA journalist mode* where we do as she says and get out of her way. She played tour guide on Capitol Hill and went about her business as if she didn't hear me say: "Check with your oncologist for breast cancer." In fact, she talked about future plans. Stell shared a life goal of empowering women to be informed about their health, opportunities, time management, education, and a plethora of topics related to a woman's well-being. Little did we know how soon she would be sharing her journey with bilateral breast cancer. Things happen for a reason.

Her phone call to me about the cancer diagnosis was devastating and heartbreaking. But as anyone who knows Stell realizes, the disbelief, numbness, and shock quickly wears off, and she goes on to the next step. She is a woman of action. I and those closest to her had been sucker punched and feeling our own vulnerability, trying to be strong and hold it together—for her. No question, no doubt that Estela would go public with her diagnosis because she had to be truthful with her audience.

"I choose to fight and I need you guys to make me laugh." Then we laughed and Team Estela assembled. We signed up for chemo buddies, surgery buddies, doctor appointment buddies, and any-kind-of-support buddies. Team Estela had drivers, people to run errands, prepare food and drink, and friends to hang out on bad and good days.

We all chose to crash the cancer party. I've seen cancer bring out the best and worst in people. It's chaotic and a time that can fly by or stand still. It takes away your peace, tests your faith and finances, and steals your time. But it can also give life, love, and renewed faith. It lets you see your value in the eyes of others. It forces you to say words that were unspoken. It forces you to find serenity. It forced me to do all those things, too.

My previous personal cancer experience was the loss of my cousin who was like a brother. He lost his battle to Non-Hodgkin's lymphoma. He was diagnosed at age 20 and died a day shy of his 21st birthday. I was 24 years old then and had lived my hardest adult experience with and through him. I have also lived the devastating effects of cancer as a physical therapist. I specialize in wound care and breast cancer lymphedema. But this time, it became personal again. I wasn't going to let Stell fight alone.

The most admirable thing I witnessed in Estela's journey was the announcement of her diagnosis on the 10:00 p.m. news. She was so regal and put together. She symbolized strength and faith that God would get her through the unknown. Not a tear rolled down her face. I recognized the fear in her voice and eyes, but she had made the choice to live, and that was that. *We* had this. *We* had her back.

As a medical care provider, I know that planning for care is integral. So, the first thing I did was get her a recliner. I knew she would need it for her surgeries, and as a comfort corner to reflect and journal her experiences. I also got her a care basket with bandages, nausea medication, an oximeter to measure oxygen levels, and chemo book and calendar to document dates and findings.

The first day of chemo was my "buddy day." This was another tough day for me as I witnessed the meds start travelling through her port-a-cath. This was real! We sat by the television and watched a recording of her announcement the night before and it was all surreal. In between calls from close friends, we filled out her FMLA, disability paperwork, made appointments with her attorney, and organized her life to put her more at ease.

Things happen for a reason. Witnessing all the calls and social media comments, I turned to her and said, "There is a purpose for why it's you. You have been a cancer advocate for thirty years. No one knows how to tell and support those stories like you. Something good must come out of all this."

And just like that, the seed for helping others less fortunate than her was planted. The Stand with Estela Fund was announced, giving Stell a sense of purpose and mission.

The third hardest day in this journey was when we took a field trip to the wig shop in Northeast El Paso. I smiled on the outside, but inside I was hurting as Stell adjusted a stocking on her scalp and tried on the wigs. In the middle of heartache was lots of laughter as she joked and played with the different colored wigs. Estela posed in all her finery. It turned into a hilarious and magical time.

I was out of town for the surgery, but I knew that next to losing her hair, the mastectomy would be the most difficult and emotional part of her journey. I prayed for her resilience, and for God to guide the hands of her surgeon. My prayers were answered, because the plastic surgeon was able to put on expanders immediately after the mastectomy, reducing the trauma of the experience for her.

Before she could move to the next surgical step—reconstruction—she needed physical therapy. I helped Stell achieve her goals quickly and was discharged with full strength and use of her arms. Reconstructive surgery, perhaps the most relaxed, joyful part of her journey, soon followed. I remember our hysterical jokes and conversations about all things related to her new breasts!

Stell has shown great strength and fortitude during her journey. I admire the way she fought and how she recovered.

Cancer brought out the best in my friend and also revealed strengths and blessings she and her family might never have recognized without it. Her thought has always been that God chose her to do His work. I believe that is true. She expressed gratitude to her family and children, but their DNA make-up is all the same: loving, positive, supportive, kind, thoughtful, humorous, and welcoming. Her family is protective, yet aware that Estela is El Paso's daughter, and she must be shared with others. Her circle of life-long friends has embraced her and rallied around her to serve their purpose in her journey.

I'm thankful that I've been able to be a navigator and sounding board. I am really glad that my smart mouth and no filter can make Stell laugh. But most importantly, it's been my privilege to share a friendship with Stell, and to be a source of comfort to her, her children, and to the rest of her family. I feel honored by the trust she placed in me, and the knowledge that God put us in each other's lives. Things happen for a reason.

TEAM ESTELA: JIMMY
MY STELL MADE ME UP MY GAME

I am a sixty-four-year-old single-minded man, who spent many years of his life singularly focused on business. People who know me say I'm tough, that I'm hard to get to know. Maybe I am, maybe I'm not.

I *do* know that I have been the captain of my ship for many years. I know the direction I want to go and I can steer myself with certainty. Yet, when Estela asked me to write about why I stayed in our relationship after learning she had breast cancer, I was surprised and lost.

The immediate answer was easy, because our relationship—even just three months old at that time—can be described in one simple yet complicated word: magical. I just knew it, felt the rightness of it then, and still do.

Stell (as I affectionately call her) and I were set up on a blind date by Toni Sides, a member of her tight circle of friends. I was quietly eating dinner alone at Koze, an Asian restaurant, when Toni tapped the back of my shoulder. I hadn't seen her in a while, so we caught up on pleasantries and each other's lives. Out of the blue, she asked if I would go out with her friend.

"I think you two would be a perfect fit," she said.

I said, "Sure, I'm always up for a good time." It's my standard line when I don't know what's going to happen. "Who is this woman you're talking about?" I asked.

Toni answered, "Estela Casas."

I knew who she was, of course. Everyone in the El Paso/Las Cruces area knows who she is! But still, when Toni walked away, I grabbed my phone and Googled her. I found a promotional ad for the Las Cruces Country Music Festival. There she was, wearing tight blue jeans, a big belt buckle, and boots, while smiling and tipping her black Stetson. My interest was piqued, and my gut told me she was special.

Shortly afterward, I found myself at brunch with Toni and Estela, in what they called their "Perfect Sunday." I was immediately drawn in by her clear and precise manner of speaking, her sense of fun and humor, her contagious laughter. And she was very easy on the eyes! My gaze followed her when she got up to go to the ladies' room. I admired the shape of her legs, visible from the pretty pink dress she wore that day. She caught me looking and smiled. I smiled right back.

Brunch lasted a couple of hours, and when things began to wind down, we decided not to let the day end there. Instead, the three of us went winery-hopping down Highway 28 toward El Paso. Our last stop was at Sombra Antigua, where a live band was playing their last set. When they finished, I remember Stell played and sang along with an Etta James song on her cell phone that seemed appropriate: "A Sunday Kind of Love."

We finished up the evening in Toni's backyard. Toni, Stell, and I shared more wine, music, and a charcuterie plate. But it was just Stell and me, two-stepping and twirling under the stars.

Stell has a way, an air about her, almost like a preacher, or a politician. Most of the time, she doesn't even truly realize this powerful influence, this charisma and charm, that draws so many to her. I didn't know if she knew that evening that she'd worked her magic on me, but it was true. I was ready to see where we might go together.

We courted over the next several weeks, slowly revealing ourselves and our lives to each other. I showed her country living, motorcycles, and the life of a cowboy. She showed me deep family connection, dancing, and music.

We had both had difficult relationships previously, so we were cautious about this one. It was two months and twelve dates before we even had our first kiss! Stell is a public figure, so we kept our evolving relationship just between us during this time. The only one who really knew what was going on was Toni, and she kept our secret.

As we continued to get closer, we began to open up more parts of our lives to each other, our inner circles. This is when I learned the fierce love, admiration, and support Stell has, not just from family, but from an entire community! As people began to become aware that we were, in fact, becoming a "we," I faced a lot of scrutiny. I heard concerns face-to-face from a lot more than just one or two people wanting to know my intentions. I felt like an eighteen-year-old boy being interviewed by a concerned and protective father on the first date.

We heard a lot of responses, including, "Go figure" or "Who would have thought?" We seem like an odd couple to outsiders. "What does he see in her?" or "What draws her to him?" Our backgrounds are vastly different, our life experiences and challenges aren't the same. Regardless of the comments, regardless of differences, I knew my own heart. And because Stell is "softer," more gentle and open than I am, I felt I knew hers too.

So, when she told me she had bilateral breast cancer, despite the shock and fear that I felt for her, I knew I wasn't going anywhere, except to North Carolina with her.

Stell and I needed to get away before starting her cancer journey. I had won a trip to Asheville, North Carolina, from Yamaha, and it would be our first out-of-town trip together.

Our first evening there was made of magic, but the next

morning showed us that cancer would keep intruding on our time. Stell had gotten a call from her oncologist. It was not what she wanted to hear (the cancer was more aggressive than they'd originally thought); it was not what she expected to hear (she would need to have chemotherapy very soon). Though she had trouble accepting what she heard, as a broadcast journalist, she had already done investigative research and had a hunch about what was ahead. She asked the tough questions and got the tough answers from her oncologist.

We needed to get our minds off the devastating diagnosis and all the "what-ifs" swirling in our heads. I had been so excited to take her to the Omni Grove Park Hotel in Asheville, and I was looking forward to the plans I had made for us. That phone call from the oncologist made all those plans seem less important, but we pushed on.

The day was cool and rainy as we ventured out. We grabbed a hotel umbrella and headed downtown to explore and eat some greasy, good, old-fashioned Southern cooking for lunch. Our Uber driver dropped us off at a touristy intersection with several restaurants to choose from. I can't remember where or what we ate, but I'm sure Stell pushed me to order something outside of my comfort zone. She has helped expand my palate. Afterward, we decided to walk off our caloric intake in the cool drizzle. We snuggled under the umbrella, seeking each other's warmth and security as we meandered up the street in silence. Both of us were still trying to digest our food (and the phone call).

It was a Thursday afternoon in Asheville, so there wasn't much activity happening on the streets. We were window shopping, peeking in at the storefronts, when I spotted a wig shop across the street. We looked at each other, crossed the street together, and walked in step together and ended up at the front steps. Together. Neither of us said a word.

Stell broke the silence in her energetic voice. "Let's go get educated!"

And we did just that.

We milled around the store, not saying much at first. Stell was curious, but clearly nervous. I felt her apprehension, anticipation, and a slight rejection, knowing she would soon be forced to slip on a wig herself.

Stell didn't want to try any of them on. "Do you like the longer one with the highlights or the shorter dark brown one?" she asked.

I smiled, but I was at a loss for words.

"Can I help you find something in particular?" asked the sales lady with a thick Asian accent.

Stell answered, "We're just looking, thank you."

I felt she didn't want to talk about her diagnosis and the reality that she would be needing a wig or two, so I spoke up. "We just learned that Estela has bilateral breast cancer and she'll be starting chemo next week. She will be losing her hair and we wanted to learn more about wigs," I said, all in one breath.

"I'm the owner, and I'm a survivor myself," she said, with a strength that seemed like it didn't fit with her small and frail appearance.

She went on to tell us how her business had been at that location for some thirty years. She had sent her daughter to college thanks to that wig shop. In her broken English, she told us she had recently received an eviction notice and had life-changing decisions to make. She had been at that location for so long and helped so many people, but the landlord did not care.

I said, "The price of progress has no compassion."

She opened up then, really starting to talk. All of her clientele were cancer patients.

"Customers first come into the shop looking like a million bucks, healthy and upbeat. But as the journey wears on, they come in to purchase a *second* wig. They are twenty pounds lighter, pale, and taking smaller steps in their gait. When they return for a third and fourth wig, they are frail and tired and shuffle with each step."

Inside my head, I completed the sentence: *They eventually stop coming when cancer beats them.*

The store owner had seen so much grief in her lifetime. She knew the types of cancers, the medicine, the chemo treatments, radiation, the successful outcomes and eventual deaths. She didn't mince words, and she didn't hold back sharing the facts she had accumulated each day inside the glass walls of her shop.

As I listened to her, I realized she probably knew more than any Doctor of Psychology, oncologist, or counselor when it came to the feelings and future Stell was now facing. She didn't speak in a surgeon's lingo; she was unfiltered, a cancer patient who was patient with my questions.

I did not talk to Stell. Stell did not talk to me. We just listened, processing the answers separately and independently of each other. It was easier that way; it was the only way we knew how to deal with what we were facing. The raw and real information hit me hard, and I needed to take in what I had just heard.

I felt sick to my stomach, got teary-eyed, and my jaw was tight.

So new in our relationship, I couldn't even start to imagine how Stell felt. I wanted to hold her and give her positive reinforcement. I didn't know what to say and couldn't find the words to tell her that she would warrior through and simply froze.

I stamped those minutes in my memory, perhaps part heart, part mind, part ignorance, sadness, sorrow, and dread. It shocked me into reality. The excursion into the shop rocked my world.

Stell didn't buy a wig that day. As we walked out, The Wig Lady said, "Good luck on your journey."

Stell's head was so full of uncertainty that she told me she didn't recall the conversation with the shop owner just moments after we left. Nothing we talked about registered; she was like a zombie. Questions flooded my mind:

What happens next?

How will my kids react to me dating a woman with cancer?

How will they cope?

How will I cope?

How will she respond to the cancer treatment?

I couldn't answer those questions, but I thought that *Stell* answering those questions could lead to her kicking me out of her life. I was told that it's common for cancer patients to feel as if they are a burden to their close friends and family. Their instinct is to push the people close to them away because they don't want to be seen sick, weak, and vulnerable. Cancer patients can become angry and don't want the people they love to see them at their worst. I accepted this as credible and noted it could happen to me.

But I knew one thing for sure.

I wasn't going to leave.

Stell's cancer journey was going to be part of *our* journey.

Stell never did push me away. Instead, she pulled me in.

When we returned to El Paso from our trip, it was just a matter of days until she began chemotherapy. You've already read here about the grace and dignity she summoned to get through it. You know about her efforts to help other women facing breast cancer, even as she was fighting for her own life.

What many of you may not know is how, after successfully navigating all the procedures, treatments, and surgeries, Stell had to come face-to-face with a second scare.

All during the healing process, Stell had to go in for checkups every three months. Sandra, one of Stell's true friends, drove her to get scheduled blood tests with her trusted doctors at Texas Oncology. It was an early morning appointment. The checkup included a cancer marker test, the CA 27.29. This test is useful in tracking any cancer activity in the body.

As they settled into the car to leave the appointment, Stell received an unexpected phone call from the nurse.

"Your cancer markers are elevated. The doctor wants you back in his office right now. You need to have a CT scan," was the message from the nurse.

It was a worst-case scenario.

Stell called me immediately. I could hear the terror in her voice, and I knew it was a distress call.

"Hi Jimmy," she said softly. "My cancer marker is up. I have to go in for a CT scan and further testing."

After that, her words were garbled. I couldn't make any sense of what she was trying to say. Sandra took over the phone, explaining the recent conversation with the oncologist's nurse.

She said, "I'm taking her in for the CT scan. We'll be at Starbucks afterward, to wait for the results. Stell says you like a caramel macchiato; should I order you a venti?"

Still reeling, I replied, "Yes, please. I'm on my way."

I dropped what I was doing and sped to Starbucks. That two-mile drive from my office was the longest and loneliest ride of my life. I opened the door to the coffee shop and saw my girl sitting across at a six-top table right next to the display where scones, cake pops, and muffins normally look appetizing. They didn't that day.

Her eyes were swollen, proof she had been crying. I gingerly snuggled in next to her, kissed the top of her head, and held her hand under the table, which is something we do often, especially when anticipating news we don't want to hear. Stell told me about her phone conversation with the nurse and shared the details of the CT scan she had just had. But in my head, I kept saying:

No, it can't be accurate.

Not again!

Why now, after eighteen months?

Why her?

In my mind, there was no way she could have a recurrence. Estela Casas was disciplined and compliant with her doctor's orders. She never skipped an appointment or treatment, ate the proper foods and drank a lot of water, and only a little bit of wine.

She stayed focused and never quit working, even though her job was very demanding. Stell got adequate sleep and never lost her faith in God. She never isolated herself or allowed herself to spiral down into a deep depression and had the best medical care available at Texas Oncology in El Paso. She was being monitored by doctors at MD Anderson in Houston.

She's a hero.

What else could she do?

Sandra and I both knew we could not let Stell slip into anger and grief. She was too emotionally fragile and the news too overwhelming. We felt helpless. Stell was in a daze.

I had been her distraction throughout her fight. This entire relationship, I tried to keep her focused on other things. We traveled together, we made new friends together, we conversed together, we laughed together and consoled each other together.

Together, together, together.

Could all the effort on her part, my part, and everyone else's part to keep her healthy have been in vain? Could the results from the CT scan show that Stell was about to lose the fight? The possibilities were terrifying. The three of us started grasping for answers and action.

"I may have to begin another round of chemotherapy . . . or maybe there's nothing doctors can do to save me," Stell said with tears in her eyes.

The possibility of the cancer metastasizing was real. These progressive cancer cells in the breast generally travel to the lungs, liver, bones, and brain. Stell had heard it all before. She knew better than us about recurrence.

That morning at Starbucks, as she and Sandra were sipping on matcha and I was drinking a caramel macchiato, Stell talked about dying with dignity or euthanasia. She told us she didn't want to be a burden and didn't want anyone to see her deteriorate if the cancer attacked her brain. Stell asked my opinion about physician-assisted suicide when living with a terminal illness.

I answered, "Why prolong the inevitable and cause unfair suffering to yourself, your family, and those who love you?"

As I said the words, I realized my statement was raw, even though it was honest. Those words are easier to express when you're only a witness, and not facing the possibility of actually carrying it through.

She contemplated her predicament, and replied, "I'm going to Portland, Oregon, so I can be euthanized where it's legal. My brother Fernando lives there, and I can die with dignity."

That statement was the nadir of her battle with cancer.

This was my breaking point.

For two hours we cried, tried to justify the cruelty of life, and comforted each other. Customers came and went. Starbucks probably turned their tables four times. Every single one of those sixty people inside the store stared at us, and some even cried with us. I would look up after concentrating like a laser beam and see all eyes on us. These patrons of Starbucks became patrons of my Stell, their Estela.

The future loomed, showing nothing but uncertainty. How would she tell her children? How would she tell her brothers and ex-husband that the cancer was back? How would we get through this?

I tried to imagine a life ahead without her, and I found that I couldn't. It was unthinkable.

Our conversation was interrupted by the ring of her cell phone. It was Dr. Valilis. Sandra and I held our breaths until we heard Stell say, "Thank you, doctor. Thank God, I was really afraid you'd call with bad news. Have a good day."

The cancer marker test had returned a false positive.

The CT scan showed no sign of cancer in Stell's body.

That day prepared us for the real possibility that cancer cells smarter than the chemo had remained. The threat is still there every day. I know it's a matter of when, not if, the cancer returns. Stell won't be declared in remission until February of 2023, and I intend to be here for that.

"Why?" she and others have asked.

Because . . .

Estela Casas, my Stell, made me up my game.

Deciding to stay in the relationship had nothing to do with her cancer journey. I wasn't going to stay involved because she was too fragile or too sick. I did not feel obligated to stay. I didn't stay because I believed she would spiral down into depression.

I stayed in the relationship because I knew, even early on, that we might have the opportunity to be meaningful partners to each other. We show respect and have admiration for one another.

Stell doesn't tell me how I, or things, ought to be; she just models that every day. She treats everyone with respect, dignity.

She is made of a different substance than any of the other women I've met and dated. Her "power of positive affirmation" makes me, and everyone around her, feel so good.

I'm not a man who lets down his guard easily. I don't really choose to let people see me. Many experiences of my life have taught me that this is the best way to stay strong and avoid being hurt. Stell doesn't play that way. She sees me, and lets me know that she sees, and that she loves what she sees.

My own children like Stell immensely. They tell me: "When I have a conversation with Estela, she is engaged. She makes me feel like she cares."

They believe she is good for me. I do too. I like to think I am good for her too.

Although Stell and I both have our own separate lives, our time together is precious and valued. We share great conversations and hold hands. We have funny little relationship rules: we always sit next to each other at the dinner table, never across from each other, so we can hold hands under the table. And when we say hello or goodbye, it always starts and ends with three kisses: one for hope, one for promise, and one for love.

She loves me for who I am. Stell lifts me up. She makes me want to be the best me I can.

We even have our own song ("Love Song" by The Cure). When I remember how that happened, it still brings a smile to my face.

It was at a surprise party for my sixtieth birthday. She sang it, wearing black cowboy boots and a wig, climbing up some steps of alfalfa bales and onto a flatbed trailer. Friends at the party were gathered by the bonfire when my friend, Skip Litt, yanked me away and toward the stage.

"Estela is on stage. Are you listening? Estela is singing to you!"
he told me.

I made my way to the edge of the stage and listened intently
to the lyrics:

"Whenever I'm alone with you
You make me feel like I am home again
Whenever I'm alone with you
You make me feel like I am whole again
Whenever I'm alone with you
You make me feel like I am young again
Whenever I'm alone with you
You make me feel like I am fun again
However far away, I will always love you
However long I stay, I will always love you
Whatever words I say, I will always love you
I will always love you."

My wish for us is that we always know the truth of these words together. I wish for Stell that she sees her son Andres graduate, not just from high school, but from college too. I wish for her the joy of helping her daughter, Carolina, pick out a wedding dress and seeing her walk down the aisle. I wish that she may witness Marcos become a Doctor of Physical Therapy.

I hope to make these wishes all come true. Together.

My Stell got to help her daughter Carolina chose a wedding dress.

Carolina looked happy and beautiful as she walked down the aisle in the dress they picked out. Stell was glowing. Marcos is now Dr. Marcos Hernandez, and Andres graduated from high school and is attending Missouri University of Science and Technology on academic and volleyball scholarships.

TEAM ESTELA: FRAN
YOUR FIGHT IS HER FIGHT TOO

When Estela asked me to work on this book with her, I experienced myriad emotions.

As a voracious news consumer, I had long admired her work, watching her every day on TV. When I entered the television news industry myself in 2002, I came to know and admire her even more as a professional, and then also as a friend. We shared many confidences and common experiences in those years. We both lost a dearly loved parent during that time. We both found ourselves the lucky recipients of later-in-life surprise babies. Besides being an important mentor for me, she provided amazing support through both blessings and challenges.

My work in that industry eventually moved me away from my hometown of El Paso. We were able to stay in touch, but certainly not to the degree we had when we were working together. In 2017, I was as shocked as everyone else to learn of Estela's breast cancer diagnosis. I'd rarely felt as powerless in my life. If I'd been in El Paso, there would have been no question that I would be on "Team Estela." I followed her journey from afar, reaching out to offer emotional support and encouragement along the way. I visited El Paso a couple of times, and I was able to meet up with Estela and see for myself how she was doing; and while I was thankful for that, I was keenly aware that I wasn't able to walk the journey with her in the way others were/could.

When Estela reached out to me to help, as she said, "Make it sing!" my first feeling was honor. Not long after, I was receiving chapter after chapter after chapter, the details of the journey that I hadn't known or experienced with her, and I felt deeply the humility of being entrusted with her story.

As we've worked our way through the editing process, I've found myself less often surprised by what I'm reading and editing, than profoundly moved by what is revealed in it. I've always known Estela to be smart, capable, strong . . . a fighter. She's also, despite being in the public eye for so many years, a very private person. The depth of her commitment to truth and education is, therefore, quite obvious in this book. The details, agonizing and brutal, touching and real, are laid bare here for everyone to see. That is courage. That is love.

I could not be prouder of Estela, or more thankful for her friendship, than I am today after having been in this labor of love with her. I hope that in reading this book, you may also know that your fight is her fight too.

Acknowledgments

This book is dedicated to my children Carolina, Marcos, and Andres.

I apologize for putting you through such a tough test. It was beyond my control.

We were all thrust into this painful journey and we have come out stronger.

We grew, together.

We grew emotionally, and didn't let our emotions get the best of us.

We grew spiritually because we turned this challenge over to God.

We grew physically, because we learned the power of a strong body through good nutrition, exercise, and proper medical care.

To Carolina, my beautiful, smart, witty, no-nonsense hospital executive daughter: you keep me grounded and humble. You spent a lot of time away from your job and money on airfare to be by our side providing structure and discipline. You are strong and bold. Thanks for reminding me to drink more alkaline water, drink less wine, get on the Peloton, and learn how to "chill." I'm working on all of the above. I can't make promises on the wine. Thanks for washing my car and organizing things around the house. You make me proud. You are my favorite daughter.

I love you with all my heart.

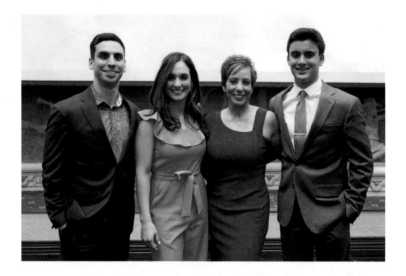

To Marcos, my light-spirited, kind-hearted son: you keep reminding me that life is too short to not enjoy the beauty in everything. All the hard work you're putting into your Doctorate of Physical Therapy is not going unnoticed and is paying off in your patients. Although I don't like how your dog EZ sheds all that hair in the house, I love her because you love her. She is still not allowed on my bed or sofas. You keep me smiling, my favorite middle son. I love you with all my heart.

To Andres, my tall, dark, and handsome son, who has been through the toughest challenges: You have blossomed into a mature young man. You have an eye on the prize, and I love you for reminding me that you still need me in your life. I love your passion for volleyball, and keep praying you grow past six feet. You're almost there! You keep me grounded, my favorite youngest son! I love you with all my heart.

To Arnoldo, we did a terrific job raising three amazing children! They are also a reflection of you. Thank you for your steadfast support and commitment to our kids.

To my brothers, Fernando and Carlos, you love me unconditionally, and I too love you unconditionally. To my sisters-in-law, Bertha and Olga, you are my blood sisters.

To Jimmy, my beloved, monogamous, adult companion. You inspire, motivate, encourage, build, and believe in me. You have helped me experience all the wonderful things life has to offer. I am forever grateful for the way you accept and embrace my idiosyncrasies and vulnerabilities. You rescued me. I love singing to you and dancing to Honeybee in the kitchen. You are my Strong and Steady.

To my sisters from another mother, Sandra, you saved my life. I am forever grateful for your unwavering friendship. You are a blessing.

Toni, your real and raw words kept me from sliding into depression. Our tango lessons also kept me sane. You are a blessing.

Patti, your good judgment, patience, persuasiveness, and ability as a reporter to be fair and balanced kept me in check. I miss our conversations in the kitchen over leftovers. You are a blessing.

Griselda, my longtime friend. Your faith in God strengthened my faith. You are a kind and gentle soul. You are a blessing.

Nicole, your quiet spirit and mischievous laughter kept me laughing. You are a blessing.

Ana, quien me ayudo a mi y a mi familia sobrellevar muchos retos eres una bendicion.

To my KVIA family, I am forever grateful for allowing me to tell my stories.

To my editor Fran, thank you for helping me bring life to my words and onto the pages in this book.

To my community, thank you for your well-wishes. There is power in prayer.